—— Praise ——

for *Exploring Sex, Love and Lust*

"*Great book on a complicated subject. I would recommend it to my patients. The best advice on finding the G spot I have read, should be part of the national curriculum.*" ~ *A Family Doctor.*

"*It is a real pleasure to see so much good and sensible advice brought together in your book. I think you did a masterful job with a lot of difficult topics. Bravo!*" ~ *A female online reader, NY.*

"*I have read a countless number of, and reviewed several, books on all aspects of 'Human Sexuality' during my career in the personal healthcare category . . . . this exciting new book from Clive Peters excels over the others . . . . readers will find it very difficult to not finish reading it in one go from cover to cover . . . .*

"*This book is a masterpiece on what can be a serious and difficult subject to cover effectively*" ~ *UK-based Medical Devices expert, and Consultant on ISO standards to Condom Mnftrs.*

"*Even though this book had a serious content , there were many humorous quotations, comparisons and illustrations that made my partner and I chuckle, leading to discussions that would otherwise have been difficult to initiate*" ~ *Dominic Finn, Dental Surgeon and Dad, England.*

"*This should be required reading for all medical students.*" ~ *A New England Physician*

"*I enjoyed reading this . . . it has a chatty and approachable style. Although accessible to a younger age group . . . is likely to appeal to older readers, too. Centred on love and respect, the book is optimistic and practical.*" ~ *Headteacher, 11-18 Community Academy, UK.*

"*It is amazing how many of the anecdotes apply to me. Had I had a copy in my youth it would have benefited me enormously. I am sure it will be widely read and benefit many.*" ~ *Chemicals Engineer, Southern England.*

"*An essential read for those young adults who wish to extend their knowledge of sexual and loving relationships. And not only them; I know a few 65 year olds who would benefit, too!*" ~ *A Family Physician, UK.*

Exploring Sex, Love and Lust

CLIVE PETERS

Edited by
Kimberly Wylie

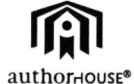

authorHOUSE®

AuthorHouse™ UK Ltd.
1663 Liberty Drive
Bloomington, IN 47403 USA
www.authorhouse.co.uk
Phone: 0800.197.4150

Editor: Kimberly Wylie
Illustrations: Sudipta DasGupta

Published by AuthorHouse 06/16/2014

ISBN: 978-1-4969-7857-8 (sc)
ISBN: 978-1-4969-7858-5 (hc)
ISBN: 978-1-4969-7859-2 (e)

By the same author:

How to Maximize Your Manhood:
What Every Red-Blooded Male Needs to Know

TO MY WIFE,

our love has never changed; it just grows deeper.

—— Disclaimer ——

The author and publisher have no responsibility for the information provided by any websites or links to websites whose address you obtain from this book. The inclusion of website addresses and links to website addresses does not constitute an endorsement by or association with us of such sites or the content, products, advertising or other materials presented on such sites. Not all websites are permanent and the author and the publisher cannot be held responsible for links to addresses or the website addresses themselves being no longer available.

—— Contents ——

—— Preface ——

So much has been written on the subject of love, but there's always been something missing, like answers to questions that are difficult to answer:

- Why do we fall in love?

- What attracts us to one person more than another?

- What makes us irresistible to some?

- What is the difference between love and lust?

- What makes good sex?

- How do we recognize and share those most intimate feelings and desires?

Then there are things no 'nice' person would dream of asking—so we carry on, in the hope 'we're doing it right.'

Nowadays, we have the Internet to seek answers and join in on forum discussions about any subject we choose. However, the uncertainty remains. Am I getting the right advice?

Recently, I was shaken to read a young woman firmly believed having sexual intercourse while standing up meant she couldn't get pregnant. Gravity apparently was on her side! That did it for me!

With the encouragement of family and many friends around the world, in many walks of life—not least the medical profession—it has been my privilege and pleasure to begin my research. Gathering the results of so many studies carried out by academics and their world-class institutions has enabled me to piece together the jigsaw that makes human relations what they are.

You now hold the result of this endeavor in your hands. I sincerely hope you enjoy and benefit from what you discover within these pages.

—— Introduction ——

"I only know that I do not know."

~Socrates

Dear Clive:

As you can tell, I have found myself quite committed of late to the idea that many men—maybe most men—really don't know all that much about women and sex. Of course, it works both ways.

Women know very little about men and frequently don't know all that much about their own bodies either. Like most people, by age 25 I thought I knew everything there was to know about sex. What a shock to learn 20 years later I knew hardly anything!

Anyway, I feel strongly that knowledge is power. That's just as true in this case as in others. I enjoy sharing what I know and have found guys seem to enjoy hearing about it. If I can help you in any way, I would be happy to.

Best,

Batwoman

Batwoman, in my estimation, is as wise as Socrates. The only difference is she is willing to share what she has learned about sex. Thanks to her willingness to share, along with many other contributors of both sexes, you'll learn more about their views in this book.

Obviously, "Batwoman" isn't her real name, but I can vouch for her authenticity and integrity. I can also promise you mind-blowing, revealing, and exciting answers to the most intimate questions from "What's going on down there?" to "I wonder if my partner is getting as much out of this as I am." to "How can I perform better?" You'll not only get answers to these questions that can sometimes be embarrassing and many more, but you'll also get the practical science behind the answers.

When we try to improve our sex lives, the first thing we think of is technique. It's only natural to want to learn the best ways to use our bodies, lips, mouths, fingers, our most sensitive spots, and even places you didn't even know you had. This is all covered in these pages.

However, to achieve amazing sex, and isn't that what we all really deserve, it is truly beneficial to also understand the science behind it—the physiology and the chemistry. These are the driving forces behind the act. We also need to understand how we communicate love and desire and how to maximize these attributes.

That's just the starting point!

Have you ever wanted to be the best lover? When we have sex, it's natural to wonder if our partner enjoys it as much as we do. We wonder if they understand our innermost desires. We wonder what they want and what we might do better—for both of us. We constantly look to please and be pleased.

For this reason, we start to ask questions of ourselves and of the opposite sex. Unlike everyday matters, however, we don't ask for advice from our parents or our best friends. Sex is perceived by many as a taboo subject—although women are better about this than men. Even if we do ask our friends for input, we're not sure they really understand what we hope to find or if their advice or experience is really applicable to us. The best person to ask, of course, is the person you're having sex with, but we often find it difficult. Within these pages, you'll discover how to get over this awkwardness.

What I am saying here is . . . Nobody's perfect, and we'd all like to do better.

This book recognizes this and recognizes we are all different.

You may have heard the expression, "Different strokes for different folks." That certainly applies to sex. When we look for answers to our most intimate questions, the first port of call is usually the Internet. If you are of a certain age, your first resource may be a periodical magazine or even a book.

The amount of information out there can be bewildering. Frequently, this information can be misleading, at best, and dishonest at worst. Where do you begin, and where do you look for answers that relate to your innermost intimate thoughts?

After you've read this book, you'll understand what drives you, what drives your partner, what's acceptable, and what's most enjoyable for both you and your partner, in an understanding and loving relationship. Yes, the best sex is within a loving relationship. In fact, the most amazing sex is between two people who give themselves completely and unreservedly to each other. Amazing sex strengthens their bond, and I believe you can continue this wonderful activity well into old age. A great sex life can even help you live longer!

There are elements to good sex that are easily identified—mutual attraction, desire and opportunity. Sex is inordinately more complex than that though.

Within these pages, you will discover how to have the best sex and how to make the most of skills you already have. You will learn from other's experiences and knowledge about our bodies—sexually speaking. You'll learn techniques to make the most of those discoveries. From the raging hormone-influenced teenage years, through the hard working mid—life years while raising a family, through the physically challenging years of later life, sex can and should be amazing. It is the glue that bonds us together.

There's no one person, male or female, who knows everything. I certainly do not claim to be in that position. However, let me share a personal experience with you.

My very first full sexual experience was in my late-teenage years. It was with a woman five years older than me. My lasting memory from this liaison was she knew a whole lot more about my body than I did! That not only astounded me, but it kicked into gear my life-long interest in wanting to learn more about sex and to constantly keep my sensual and sexual skills at their peak.

Why would I share this with you? For this book to be of value to you, you and I need to believe in the same objective—a desire to have the best sex possible. If you've read this far, I'm sure we are on the same wavelength.

Allow me to use a driving analogy.

You can get behind the wheel of a car, and the more miles you drive, the more skilled you become. However, we all run into a problem from time-to-time. From unintentionally driving the wrong way on a one—way street to running out of fuel, it happens to the best of us. If something mechanical or electrical breaks down, we go to a mechanic to put it right. Sadly, there's nobody like that in our bedroom!

Sure, we can call our family physician or a specialist, like a gynecologist or urologist, for advice or a cure if the problem requires medical attention, but where can we learn what the best lovers do? How can we anticipate problems and either avoid or overcome them without discussing them with our dubiously knowledgeable friends?

This is where the experts have the answers. Their multitude of studies and surveys, in all things sexual, bring the science and solutions to our aid. In my research, I have made friends with many highly-qualified and communicative professionals of both sexes who have helped me put this book together. When things aren't quite right, we look for answers. This is how I began a journey of discovery about sex and all its driving forces. Through these pages, you can share this journey with me.

As I've said before, we're all different. This theme runs throughout this book. As an example, not everyone wants to learn about anal sex, and that's understandable. In case you might be curious though, this topic and many other sexual activities are covered.

You may already enjoy oral sex, cunnilingus and/or fellatio, (better known by many as "giving head" or "giving a blow job"), but it's always worth listening to how other people have increased their skills and how both partners can heighten their enjoyment.

It goes without saying, the female orgasm is a fascinating subject. By the end of this book, you will discover the many ways female orgasm can be achieved, the difference between clitoral and vaginal orgasm, and how to stimulate each. You'll even learn how to work up to female ejaculation—better known as squirting. Every woman can give a different description of how an orgasm feels.

As we go through life, our circumstances change—physiologically, psychologically and sexually—and not always for the better.

Recognizing where you are in this scenario is key. Knowing you're not alone and your perceived problem is usually a lot more common than you thought really helps. Take premature ejaculation (cumming too quickly) as an example. You will read how this originated and ways to take control over peaking too soon. Erectile dysfunction, also known as ED, (the inability to get or maintain a hard erection) is a problem that affects all men at some time in their life, which results in disappointment and frustration. It can even lead to the break-up of relationships. The warning signs and situations that lead to ED are described, and solutions are provided beyond simply Viagra!

Size is discussed, along with the opinions of men and women on the topic of size. If a man wants to increase his size, guidelines are given, along with options on how to increase your size. In regards to women, we discuss breasts and their size and shape, as well as what surveys show about our feelings about them.

We talk about nipples, vulvas, the clitoris, labia, vaginas, and body hair. Penises, large and small, testicles and scrotum, and the volume of semen are also discussed in detail. This book is no holds barred on all topics concerning sex. A description of the G-spot and how to stimulate it, as well as the location of the A-spot and three ways to reach it, are described.

The presence and use of pornography is discussed, including its effect on us and its pros and cons. You'll read about communication and the part hormones play in our desires, actions and reactions. You'll learn how to develop skills in conveying what you desire and triggering those same desires in your partner, from how to use your eyes to how to say the right things to touch and smell. We'll even introduce you to cyberspace!

You'll learn how to develop those muscles to keep us in good physical shape for sex and how to keep it up well into old age. You'll discover the best positions for maximum penetration, stimulation or pure enjoyment, depending on your age, location and opportunity. Whether you're just beginning to build your sexual history, busy raising a family or in the golden years of retirement, you'll learn the hows and whys of the best sex for every stage of your life. From mutual masturbation to full—blown sex, this book will have the sexual revelation you've been seeking!

I never intended this to be a sex manual, even though there will be those who might refer to it as such. It is more of a collection of thoughts, ideas and shared experiences between men and women, of all ages. Everyone from universities to individual doctors to professors report on their findings of their studies on human behavioral and sexual activities. Reports of the many medical studies, from around the world, abound in these pages. Because of the very private and personal nature of comments made by contributors, their names, or true names, may not appear, except for those who have given permission or who have previously published papers on sex-related subjects. These are given their proper accreditation. There are comments made by famous personalities drawn from their published views on sex you will recognize, and their names do appear.

That's enough of the teasing and hints of what's to follow. Turn the page and we will begin our journey.

—— 1 ——
In the Beginning

*Find a guy who calls you beautiful instead of hot, who calls
you back when you hang up on him, who will lie under the stars
and listen to your heartbeat, or will stay awake just to watch
you sleep . . . wait for the boy who kisses your forehead, who
wants to show you off to the world when you are in sweats, who
holds your hand in front of his friends, who thinks you're just
as pretty without makeup on. One who is constantly reminding
you of how much he cares and how lucky he is to have you . . . .
The one who turns to his friends and says, "That's her.'*

~Love Quotes, Facebook—Nino Rostomashvili

We all start off in this life as virgins. As we grow up, we are
exposed to new experiences we can learn and benefit from, allowing
us to enjoy our lives and the people around us. We want to be
confident—especially with those we fall in love with. However,
when it comes to sex, where do we begin to learn?

From our parents?
From our teachers?

No, most often it's from our peers—the least experienced and
knowledgeable people around us!

True sexual relationships are typically left for us to discover on our own. Yes, you can say there are plenty of books available on this subject. You can point out there's plenty to see and hear, as well as read, on the Internet. However, no written word, or explicit sex video or photograph, can teach you about the thrill of falling in love or the rush of feelings coursing through your veins when you are joined as one with the naked body of the person you care about. It can't tell you how you should behave, so both of you can reach the dizzying heights your friends brag about.

For reasons you will begin to learn for yourself, learning how to make love is not a subject our parents or teachers really want to talk about. Being shy about what you get up to between the sheets or feeling the topic is inappropriate are just two of the simple reasons your father and mother may choose not to broach the subject.

Your closest friends might talk about their experiences when you ask them, but as each one recalls only experiences relevant to their own desires and fantasies—or those they do not enjoy—the relevance to your own life may be totally different. How will you know? It is this difference that makes people reticent about talking about sex. They don't want to be seen or heard as *different*, or risk upsetting someone else with their experiences or views.

The First Time

Confidence comes with experience, but no matter how confident you might be, the very first time you realize the opportunity for sex presents itself, and you're about to share the most intimate physical experience of your life, anxiety often takes a hold on you. This happens to a lot of people. It is one of my main reasons for writing this book, so you know what to expect and to understand what is going on in your mind and body.

To assure you you're not alone and to illustrate the point, here are two true stories—one from a man and one from a woman. Don't be surprised by either of them. Their experiences are more common than you may think. Only the names are fictitious.

Adam's Story

This story was shared with me, by Jason Julius of Orgasmarts. com:

I'm not a particularly good looking fellow, and never managed to attract any girls in high school, but I definitely found girls attractive. I would dream about a certain girl I would have loved to get real close to. I would toss myself off to sleep thinking about her.

In college, the girls shared dormitories, and there was one particular girl I really fancied. She shared her room with another student. One day, out of the blue, the girl I fancied came up to me and told me her roommate had left for a few days vacation. She asked if I would like to come up and have supper with her.

You could have knocked me down with a feather! I had no idea she liked me at all, let alone wanted to spend an evening together—alone in her room. **Never give up on yourself***, I told myself with a smile.*

That evening I arrived, with a bottle of wine, freshly shaved and showered and wearing my best casual clothes. We ate and drank, talked, smiled, and laughed a lot, and it became evidently clear she wanted to take me to bed. While she disappeared into the bathroom, I took off my clothes but dived beneath the duvet to take off my underpants—I was that shy, and I didn't want her to see how small my dick was.

She came back into the room and asked what was I doing underneath the covers. I replied, "Putting on a condom."

In fact, I was actually trying to get an erection! No matter how hard I tried my favorite friend refused to get up. Putting on a condom was out of the question until I was erect.

Anxiety had taken hold. The more I tried the worse it got—just a limp dick. She suggested, as she was on the pill, we might do it without bothering with the condom. This woman was so sympathetic, so kind, so lovely, and I was being an absolute failure. She patiently took my penis in her hand and gently persuaded it into a semi-erection.

Impatient to get going, but still with a slightly limp penis, I managed to literally stuff it into her vagina. No sooner was I there in that beautiful wet, warm place, and with all the effort having gone before, I felt my semen rising—there was nothing I could do to stop it.

My humiliation was complete.

Eve's Story

I'm 18 and have never had a boyfriend, as I haven't felt ready. I would now like a relationship, though I'm not ready to have sex. I desperately need more sexual knowledge. I know nothing about the male anatomy and little about my own. My mother would be uncomfortable giving me sexual advice, and I'd feel embarrassed asking my friends. Are there any books I could read or is this something I can only learn through experience?'

Eve's story came as an e-mail to me and tells of the torment some women go through even before getting close to a man. Eve was brave enough to recognize her own situation and ask for help in overcoming her natural anxiety.

There are numerous stories by other women, some reminiscing with warm feelings about a fleeting relationship and others about the first step in a lifetime's partnership. Still more describing their disappointment.

Why was it so quick?

When can I expect to have an orgasm?

Am I so unattractive that he had to leave early?

Why do my friends tell me it is so wonderful when my experience tells me I'd rather enjoy a soak in the tub with a good book?!

Love isn't all about sex, but it does play a huge part in keeping the flame burning. To begin with, the best advice is to get to know each other first. Consummation is an old-fashioned word that used to apply to a marriage. In other words, you were not expected to sleep with each other until after you were married. This virginal expectation is now outdated for most, but the logic behind the reasoning still applies. Sex is better when it is part of a loving relationship. It's better not to be pushed into having sex before you're ready.

If a man cares about a woman, he will take time to get to know the woman—just kiss and touch until she feels ready to take things further. Sex is natural, but everyone is inexperienced at first. The nice thing about making love with someone special is learning together what you both enjoy. When this stage is reached, you can both further your understanding of each other's bodies, desires and fantasies by delving into the pages of this book.

—— 2 ——
Are You Obsessed With Sex?

Good girls go to heaven; bad girls go everywhere.

~ Helen Gurley Brown

It's February 14th, St. Valentine's Day. In the balmy evening air, a young couple strolls arms around each other's waists along the beach. We're in Gran Canaria, one of a small group of islands just north of the Tropic of Cancer and 80 miles off the West Coast of Africa. The couple pauses for a moment, looks lovingly into each other's eyes and enjoys a lingering kiss, as the sound of the surf lapping the sand provides a romantic musical background.

My wife and I smile knowingly at each other, while we watch this demonstration of love and other emotions for all to see. We have a good feeling about what will happen next!

It's easy to argue nowadays that we, as a society, are generally obsessed with sex. I'm guessing if you are a male reading this book, you've probably been told at least once in your life, "It's all you ever think about!" I think that's a little unreasonable.

We've all joked about how a man only wants to move in with his girl, so he can get more sex. And, she only agrees to let him move in, because she sees it as a move toward marriage. I have news for the gentlemen—and they won't necessarily like it—a study, published in the *Journal of Family Issues*, showed men and women agree on many benefits of moving in together. However, Professor Penelope Huang, who led the research, said, "The notion that cohabitation allows for more frequent opportunities for sex, compared to dating, was emphasized much more by the men in our study than the women.[1]

"Men also linked living together far less strongly to marriage than women. They tended to view it as a 'test drive,' without specific connections to marriage, whereas women tended to discuss it as a short interval on the way to marrying their partner," according to Professor Huang.[2]

Professor Huang, and other researchers from the University of California Hastings in San Francisco, questioned approximately 200 men and women in their late 20s on reasons for and against moving in with a partner. Women volunteered love as a reason to live together three times as often as men. However, men mentioned sex four times more often than the women.

Dr Pauline Rennie-Peyton, a psychologist specializing in relationship problems, said, "Living with someone is not necessarily a commitment. If women think it's a stepping stone to marriage, then they need to be clear about it from the beginning.[3]

Man and woman were put on this earth to procreate. To do so, we must do what comes naturally—have coital sex. OK, that's a bit formal, but we all know what we're talking about here. To use the vernacular: screwing, dipping your wick, shagging, fucking, having it away. My generation called it 'making love'—to my mind, a much more romantic and all-encompassing expression. Call it what you like, as long as you know what we're talking about. My hope is that by the time you've absorbed the contents of these pages, you'll understand the question—are you obsessed with sex—as well as have the answer!

The Best Sex

Over the years, we have learned the best sex is always preceded by love and emotion. These feelings bind us together. This is the natural drive that make us select a partner, desire to settle down and raise a family. Research of all things 'penile,' in recent years, has uncovered a plethora of interesting facts relating to this drive. This includes the chemistry going on in our minds and bodies that creates these desires and how they control our feelings and emotions. With this knowledge, it should be possible to enhance every aspect of sex and deepen our understanding of each other's needs, as well as our differences.

Humans are one of the rare species that have been blessed with the necessary parts to make sex pleasurable. With contraception available to all, we are free to enjoy the act and freed from the primary purpose of sex—procreation. Sex can be recreational, and I firmly believe that good and frequent sex not only helps keep you in good physical shape, it can also extend your life.

Sharing My Findings with You

As I've mentioned, I'm not a doctor, but I have lived a long and sexually active life (and stayed together with the same woman for over 50 years—so I must have been doing something right!).

When things aren't quite right, we look for solutions. This is how I began a journey of discovery about sex and all its driving forces and started writing about it. Because of the nature of very private sexual experiences, many correspondents have asked that I maintain their anonymity and attach a pseudonym to their contribution—even professional people who don't wish to be named in order to save embarrassment to their friends and family. However, don't let this detract from the verity of my findings written in this book. Perhaps I should mention, if you are sensitive about seeing pictures of naked bodies—including close-up illustrations of penises and vaginas—you should turn the pages of this text cautiously.

I hope you agree it is a good idea to start with the basics. Since early childhood, we've all been interested in both our own genitalia and that of the opposite sex—so we'll begin there.

—— 3 ——
Anatomy 101

Anatomy is to physiology as geography is to history;
it describes the theatre of events.

~Jean Francois Fernel

It's important to know how the penis and vagina function and how they're constructed. You need to understand the hydraulic actions that make the penis hard and erect, as well as the processes behind what makes the vagina wet, if you want to expand your knowledge about sex and how to have amazing sex. As Fernel notes in his quote on anatomy above, this is the theater of your sexual events!

Male Genitalia

External Male Anatomy

In the unexcited, flaccid state, the penis hangs outside the body with a sack, called the scrotum, hanging beneath it. The head (*glans*) of the penis has a hole through which urine passes, as well as seminal fluid when orgasmic. 'Glans' is Latin for acorn. If you're looking at the end of a penis, with the foreskin just allowing the head to show through, it does bear some resemblance to an acorn.

Figure 1: Male Anatomy External View

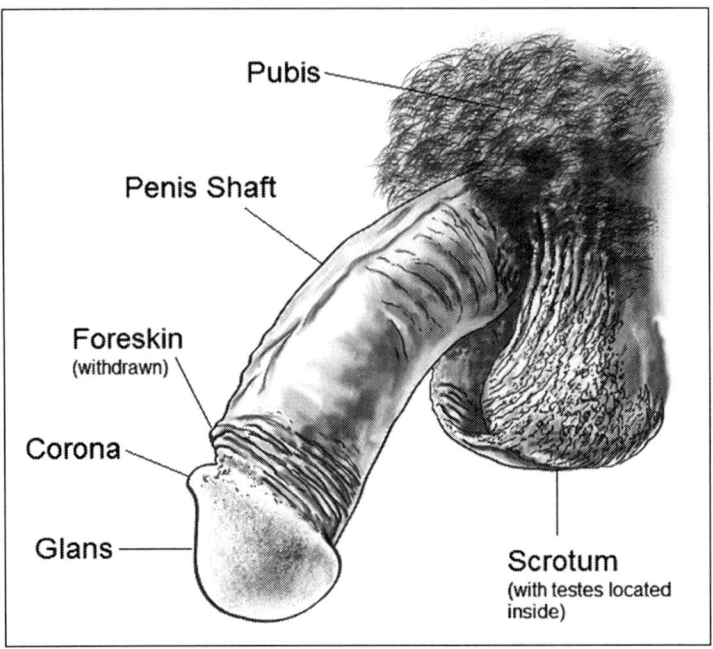

As the human form evolved, fortunately so did the penis! Early man had spikes on his penis to remove the sperm of others who had mated with a female, so his semen would be implanted instead of the other male. Thankfully, as we evolved to become monogamous, the spikes disappeared. Interestingly, the coronal rim, around the base of the head, is all that is left of that inherited shape.

The foreskin covers the shaft. It is capable of being rolled over the glans to protect it while the penis is flaccid and rolls back to expose the head when entering a vagina or masturbating. For health or religious reasons, some men are circumcised. This means sufficient foreskin has been removed, so the glans remains exposed whether flaccid or erect. This is sometimes referred to as being 'cut' or 'uncut.' Contrary to what you might think, there is little to no difference in sensitivity between cut and uncut men.

The scrotum, the bag with the wrinkly skin, holds the testes (plural of testicle). This is where sperm is continually produced, in a myriad of tubes. When mature, the sperm is held in one long tube called the *epididymis*. Testosterone, the male hormone, is also produced by cells within the testes. Now, let's talk about the male parts you can't see.

Internal Male Anatomy

The urethra is the tube that ends at the tip of the penis. The exit point is called the *meatus*. The urethra connects to the bladder, which stores urine until the man is ready to expel it. Situated underneath the bladder, at the point where it joins the urethra, is the prostate gland.

Figure 2: Cross-section Internal Male Anatomy

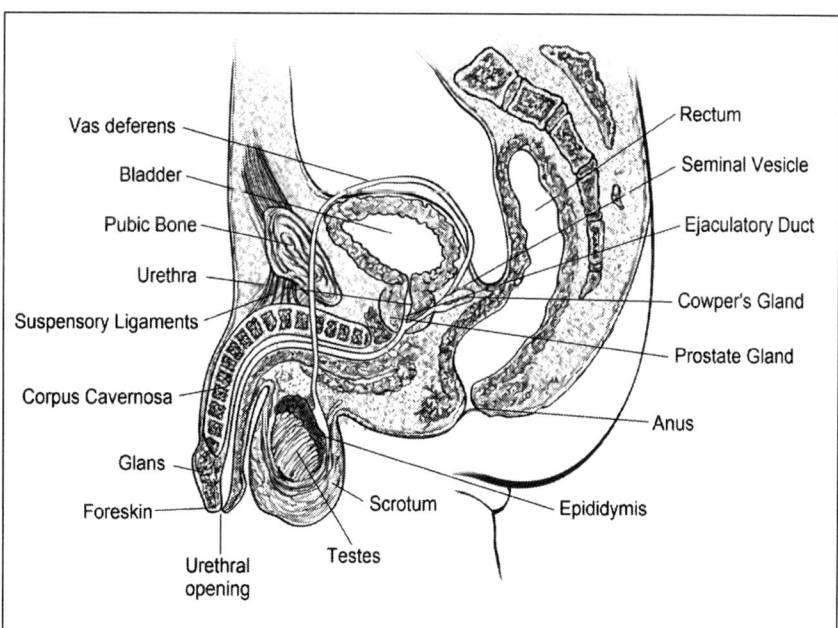

The prostate is shaped a little bit like a doughnut and is roughly the size of a walnut. The urethra passes through the hole in the middle of the prostate. This gland, along with the seminal vesicle, produces the fluid that carries sperm from the male body when a man ejaculates.

Sperm are carried through a small tube, called the *vas deferens,* that travels from each testicle to the prostate. It is these tubes that are severed if a man undergoes a vasectomy. A vasectomy is a male contraceptive surgical procedure and is sometimes referred to as 'the snip' (More information on the vasectomy process can be found in Chapter 22—Conception and Contraception).

There's one more gland we need to cover in this section—the Cowper's gland. This gland creates a lubricating liquid to help the flow of sperm along all of these tubes, as well as provides a safe saline environment for them to travel in. This is the clear liquid, rather like very fine syrup, that sometimes appears at the tip of the penis before ejaculation.

Male Hydraulics

A man's penis becomes erect thanks to the wonders of hydraulics. When stimulated by touch, sight, smell, or whatever turns him on, the brain sends a signal along the nerves to open up the arteries that feed blood into the penis. Blood flows at an increased pressure, up to ten times its normal rate, into the two major blood vessels that run the length of the penis shaft.

The *corpora cavernosa,* as they are called, expand against the surrounding *corpus spongiosum,* making the whole shaft rigid. The penile veins that would normally allow the blood to flow back out of the penis are effectively squeezed shut by this action, thus retaining the extra blood in the corpora cavernosa until another signal is sent down through the nervous system to tell the arterial blood vessels to ease up on the additional pressure. This signal is sent automatically following ejaculation.

The Physiology of an Erection

If the foregoing was all that was involved in an erection, the penis would swell but would remain hanging down. Penetrating a vagina would have to be assisted, because there would be nothing to stop the penis from wiggling around like a limb hanging on by its skin. Ligaments running the length of the penis and anchored within the body provide the tension required against the blood-engorged penis, to make it stand up and out. More about how this works in a moment. We are now getting to the parts that not only control the rigidity of the penis and make it erect without assistance but also those same parts that stretch and allow the penis to grow in length and width, under the pressure of the increased blood flow.

Figure 3: Penis Shaft Cross Section

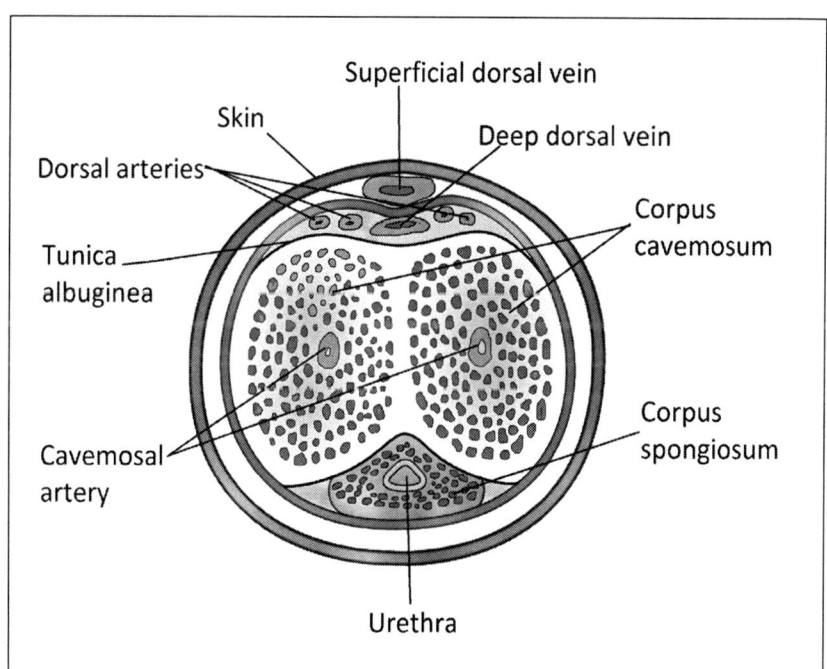

Surrounding these blood vessels is a tough, rubber-like mass that forms the wall of resistance to the extra blood pressure and makes it rigid. These tissues, referred to as the *tunica*, extend from just behind the glans to a point close to the anus. When considering the full length of the tunica, the penis is actually considerably longer than most people think! This area where the tunica extends to is what can be felt at a point halfway between the scrotum and anus. Known as the perineum, this is an erotic pressure point, especially when the shaft is engorged with blood.

Close to the prostate, the tunica is attached to the pubic bone by ligaments. These ligaments resemble a bundle of strings reaching from the underside of the glans back to the pubic bone. At each end, they fan out to provide a secure anchorage. These ligaments comprise long and short, thick and thin, lengths to make up the whole ligamentous attachment.

For the sake of comparison, imagine the penis as the boom of a crane. The vertical section from which the boom swings horizontally is the body. The ligaments are attached to the vertical section at a point above the boom and extend nearly to the end of the boom. You can imagine what would happen if you were to cut those ligaments (the procedure followed by those who want their penis surgically extended.) The boom—the penis—would have nothing to hold it up!

With nothing to hold it back, all that tunica slips forward a couple of inches, making the penis that much longer. However, it would need to be lifted by hand and guided into the vagina, without the ligament support. Even then, the man does not have the control by body movement he normally has, because his penis is no longer anchored where it is needed. It's one of the reasons I am not a fan of this surgery.

Incidentally, the increase in penis length during an erection can vary from one man to another. We are all different! It can range from less than a quarter of an inch to 3.5 inches. Shorter penises tend to gain about twice as much length as longer ones when erect.[4]

Female Genitalia

External Female Anatomy

The following illustration shows a female, lying on her back, legs spread and as if she were gently spreading her *labia majora* to give a clearer view, to show the component parts of the vulva. For the sake of clarity, pubic hair is not shown.

If you're a woman and thinking "Mine doesn't look like that!" don't worry. Remember, we're all different! This includes what our sex organs look like. The point of the illustration below is to identify the various parts. This way you'll not only know where each part is located, but you'll recognize each part when you see it.

For a woman to have a similar view, she could squat over a mirror and gently part her labia with her fingers. In this way, you can expose all of the inner parts we have identified in the illustration following.

Starting at the top of the Figure 4, we can see the *Mons Pubis,* sometimes referred to as Venus's Mount. This is often naturally covered by pubic hair; however, as noted, in our illustration we have removed the pubic hair, in order to give you the clearest view possible of the vulva. The Mons Pubis then separates into two folds of skin, called the *labia majora* and *labia minora.*

Nestled in between them, at the top of the separation, is the clitoris, covered by a hood of skin. A man has more nerve endings in his feet than in his penis. There are 4,000 nerve fibers in a penis compared with 7,000 in one foot. In contrast, A woman's clitoris has 8,000 nerve endings.

When I was a kid and my mother cooked chicken for dinner, she would save the breastbone from the carcass and gently dry it out in the oven. This then became a 'wishbone,' which two people could tug apart using only their little fingers until the now brittle bone snapped. Whoever ended up with the larger piece was allowed a secret wish.

Figure 4: Vulva Anatomical Drawing

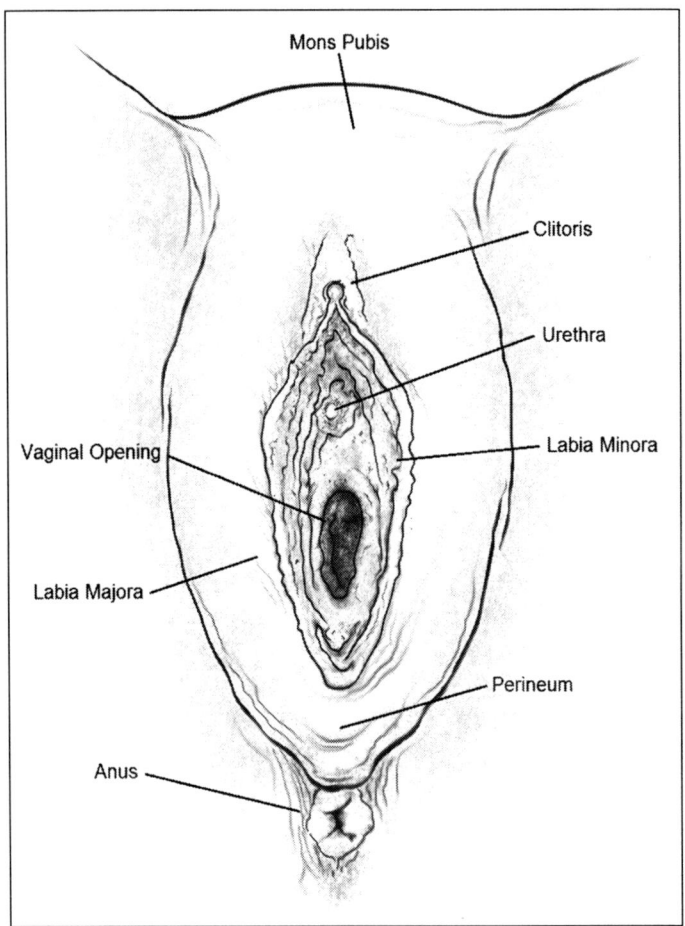

Why am I telling you this? Simple! Hold up a wishbone, with its joint at the top, and you are looking at the same configuration as the female clitoris—only the clitoris is not made of bone! Instead, it is formed of the same materials as the male penis. It has a glans head, corpora cavernosa and corpus spongiosum, but no urethra.

Instead of a foreskin, the clitoris is protected by a skin hood. The wishbone-shaped 'legs' carry the same tissues and nerves down along either side of the vulva. Despite its relatively small size, the clitoris has as many nerve endings as a penis. Knowing this concentration of nerves should help you appreciate its delicate sensitivity!

The clitoris and the outer third of the vulva share a common nerve—the *pudendal* nerve. There's also a small nerve called the dorsal nerve of the clitoris (DNC). This is the main nerve associated with orgasm in the female. Each individual's network of nerves is unique to them—just like fingerprints. We really are all different!

Immediately below the clitoris is the opening to the urethra. It is through this opening urine passes. Below the urethra, as you can see in the illustration of the spread vulva, you see the opening to the vagina protected by two sets of 'lips'—the inner being the labia minora and the outer the labia majora.

The outer labia are the equivalent of what's left of the male scrotum. These act as doors to the vagina and protect the inner labia. The outer labia also provide resistance to the foreskin of an uncircumcised penis, thus rolling it back as the penis enters the inner labial area, which is lubricated in the aroused female by the Bartholin's glands.

These lips also carry sensitive nerves and blood vessels that swell the lips, increasing pleasure for the female and making easier passage for penetration when stimulated. The area posterior to the opening to the vagina, where the outer labia meet at their lower end and the anus, is the perineum—yet another area for sexual stimulation.

The Hymen

What you can't see in the illustrations above is the hymen. Nobody really knows the purpose of a hymen, but it is a rare film of skin partially covering the opening to the vagina in virgins. I say rare because most women unintentionally break their hymen at a very young age, through sports or exercise, or through the use of tampons.

If you are female and have never had penetrative sex, please be reassured even in the event your hymen is still intact, a caring first lover should cause little or no pain. Please ignore stories of horrendous bleeding. A completely intact hymen will produce only a few specks of blood when broken, and this happens only once. This is another reason for choosing carefully your first sexual partner; it's a special event in every woman's life!

Female Internal Sex Organs

Figure 5: Cross-Section Female Reproductive System

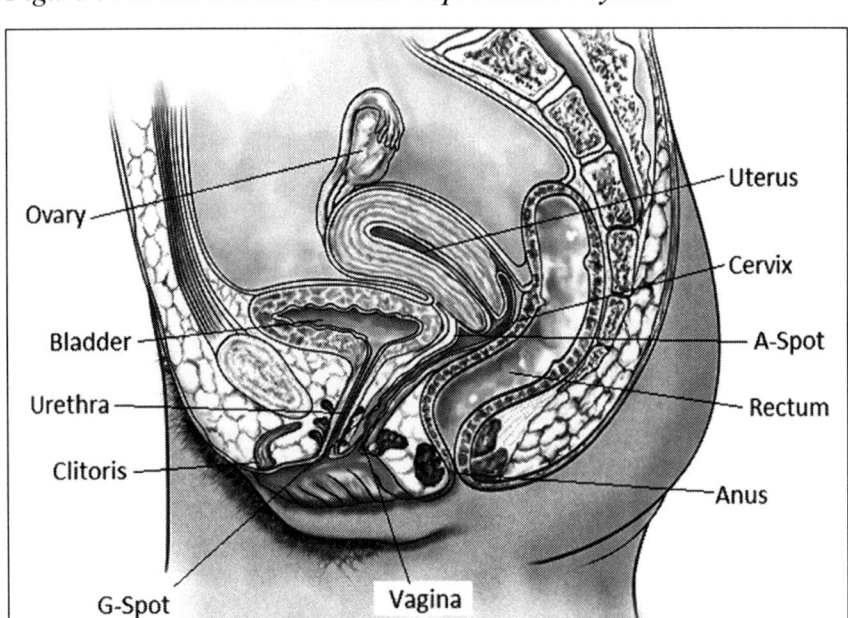

Female Genitalia Terminology

Before we go any further, the medically descriptive terms are beginning to stack up. To make sure we're on the same wavelength, and to put it in the vernacular once more, we're describing pussy, hoo-ha, vag, muff or minge, here. There are less-than-attractive names used to describe that warm and inviting place. However, a common mistake is the use of 'vagina' where the word 'vulva' would be correct.

The vulva refers to the visible external sexual organs of the female. The vagina is the canal whose entrance is situated within the vulva and ends inside the body at the cervix—the entrance to the uterus, or womb. No studies have been made on the average length of a vagina, but in its unexcited state the length is considered to be about 4 inches (10cms). Just like men's penises, vaginal length varies from woman-to-woman.

We'll talk more about the vagina and the elusive and mysterious (and sometimes thought of as mythical) G-spot in Chapter 9—The Female Orgasm.

— 4 —

The Penis

God gave men a penis and a brain, but unfortunately not enough blood supply to run both at the same time.

~ Robin Williams.

When deciding on a title for this section, I first called it "Your Penis" but thought it might put the ladies off reading this chapter. I then thought about calling it "His Penis," thinking it would attract the attention of the ladies. Finally, I chose "The Penis," because the penis is clearly of interest and importance to both genders, albeit sometimes for different reasons.

What Women Think When They See A Penis

Let's kick off with a discussion of a few impromptu studies conducted to discover the answer to a question most men wonder about. Knowing men are often fixated on their penis size, contributors to several online publications reached out to women to learn what really goes through their minds when they see a man's penis for the very first time. The responses these surveys received were quite enlightening!

One woman responded that, despite the common belief a longer penis was what women wanted, she always looked for girth. The respondent stated, "For me, width is way more important than length. Even if he's got a short penis, if he's really thick, I get really excited about sleeping with him."[5]

Some women who responded were more practical—checking out a partner for the first time for any signs of sexually transmitted diseases. As one woman noted, "If I'm playing with his balls with my hands and getting him hard, I'm probably also using that as an opportunity to check for any sores, bumps, scabs, etc. just to be safe."[6]

Color variations of the penis are sometimes a surprise to women. One woman from a *Cosmopolitan* survey described a past lover as having a "neapolitan dick," which was a light tan around the base, very dark just before the glans, and completed with a very pink head.[7] Despite the tri—color effect, she recalled enjoying this particular penis very much. A respondent to a similar survey conducted by *Men's Fitness* also was surprised by a lover's coloring. She noted, "I've never seen that shade of purple on a human being before . . . but the color was just another sign of extreme arousal, so yes, it made a difference. In the best possible way."[8]

Most women, however, are just happy to see a penis. Responses included:

- "Penises are really quite fascinating. Because I don't have one, I just want to look at my partners'—regardless of size, shape or color!"[9]

- "Chances are if I am seeing your penis it's because I actually like you, so when I first see it, it's this kind of anxious moment when I'm conscious of actually holding my breath—because there's a small risk I might not like it. Then again, I'm not super picky. I mean, I'm willing to work with you here."[10]

- "One boyfriend seemed almost embarrassed that his penis was just average size, and wouldn't ever let me compliment how much I liked it. But I wasn't lying—it felt amazing! Guys: When a woman let's you know how much she loves your package, take the compliment . . . she probably means it!"[11]

Nicole Beland, contributor to *Men's Health* magazine, isn't looking for size either, as her first thought when seeing a new penis. Instead, she's looking for hardness. Beland notes,

> *The first thing I notice isn't size, but solidity. Any sign of softness, of semierect indecision, feels like a personal insult. He must not want me. A penis that's as rigid as a flexed biceps, on the other hand, fills me with the confidence of a dominatrix and the enthusiasm of a high school cheerleader. It also triggers an involuntary response between my legs.*[12]

Even women who admitted to assessing the size of a guy's package when she gets a first look weren't nearly as hard to please as many men fear. "First, I assess his size, but not in a judgmental way. Just a casual comparison to past partners. As long as it's proportionate to his body, it doesn't matter,"[13] one woman responded. In the end, most women concluded it wasn't the size of the penis, but rather what the man did with it that determined if they remembered it fondly.

Penis Topics

I ran a blog for a few years, to support and encourage (male) readers of my book, *How to Maximize Your Manhood—What Every Red—Blooded Male Needs to Know.* I always started my posts with a heading, so potential readers could pick out subject matter that interested them or move on to other things.

Software allowed me to analyze the number of hits, for specific topics, as well as a mountain of other information but not the identity of the interested parties. It did, however, under the cloak of anonymity, allow an exchange of views to be seen.

Apart from matters of size, which I will come to in a moment, the two most significant things I found were:

1. The greatest number of hits of all time were made on February 15th (the day after Valentine's Day), and

2. The post that attracted the most hits, and comments, was headed: 'Harder Erections, Greater Control, More Ejaculate.'

This didn't surprise me, but what did was the interest shown in this topic by females. Guys, there are women out there who want to help their man. They know it's very much in their best interest to have a partner who's confidence is built and maintained, by having a healthy and strong performing penis!

Does Size Matter?

As noted, the number one penis topic on guys' minds is—Does size matter? We hear sayings like, "It's not the size of the boat; it's the motion of the ocean that matters." However, men still wonder—is that true, or is that just some saying an inadequately-sized man came up with to make himself feel better? If a guy's seen male porn stars, it's enough to make even well-endowed men feel insecure about their penis size!

Instead of listening to adages or comparing a penis to one in a movie, let's listen to at what a real woman has to say on the topic of how important penis size really is to her. When asked what she thinks about size, here's what Batwoman had to say:

> I don't care about cock size. What I care about is love, passion, sexual curiosity, lust, communication, mutual exploration, openness, shared fantasies, and lots of hot sex. How big he is, is not nearly as important as who he is, how we feel about each other, and how much fire there is between us. Do I want my lover to be skilled in bed? Absolutely. Do

I want him to get hot and hard for me and be able to satisfy me? Absolutely. Does cock size play a role in that? Nope.

For me, what matters is the guy—not the size of his member. If he turns me on, treats me well, and can please me in bed, I would not care if he was on the smallish end of cock size. Why? Because I can (and have) had GREAT sex and GREAT orgasms with guys that had smallish cocks. It really, truly is all about chemistry between me and a guy, and how he uses what he has. I keep saying that over and over, but I'm afraid that most guys don't believe it.

Much more important than cock size is lovemaking technique—patience, knowing about a lady's body and how to excite her and bring her to orgasm in different ways. EQ (erection quality) and self-control play into this too. I like an adventuresome lover with a sense of humor, a man who is willing to try new things to please me and to encourage me to try new things to please him. I want long, sexy lovemaking sessions, where we both use our hands and mouths all over each other, and lots of oral sex (both ways). I want him to love to look at my body and stroke me, and sometimes bring me to orgasm with his fingers. When we get to intercourse, I want it to last a while and I don't want it to be in the same position every time. I want to feel passion and urgency sometimes, patience and humor at other times. That's a long list, right? And—gasp—cock size isn't even on it.

So, where does cock size fit in? For me, it is something like a "bonus added" feature. If you are larger, maybe it makes some things feel a bit nicer, maybe it makes some positions easier . . . . and that would be great. But it is totally NOT the main thing I am shopping for in a man or even really on the list of essentials at all.

Reassurance

Gentlemen, if that doesn't reassure you I'm not sure anything will!

Having said this, I would admit to being appalled at a friend's confidential admission that when making love to his girlfriend one day she asked, "Is it in yet?" I can only guess how damaging an innocent question must have been to his ego, let alone his confidence! You would not be surprised to hear he subsequently spent a lot of time working to do something about the size of his penis.

For a man, his perceived problem can be he thinks the size of his penis is directly in proportion to his attractiveness to women, even though the size of his manhood is always hidden by his clothing. However, if he does have a large penis in his pants, it gives him confidence. Put simply, find me a well-endowed man, and I will show you a confident one.

For the average man, he thinks the bigger his penis, the better he will feel about himself. Apart from that, there's no logical reason for wanting a bigger penis. He might be disappointed to hear in order to procreate, and even give pleasure in the sexual act:

Size does not matter.

As a man, you may find this difficult to accept. The man with the larger penis has always been the envy of his friends. Isn't that right? Well, maybe. If so, why? Man doesn't know the answer; all he knows is he thinks he'd be more confident, not just in bed but also in everything else he does in his life.

Men don't talk about these things. There's something in the male psyche that makes it difficult for him to broach the subject. He'll ignore it as long as he can get away with giving the impression to his peers everything is fine in the trouser department and the size of his genitals leave nothing to be desired.

Urologists will tell you they are frequently asked if there is a way to increase penis size. Why wish for a larger penis though? What brings on the desire to do something about a man's size? One thing is certain: We're all different!

Take a look at this informative website, TargetMap.com, to see just how different we can all be. Looking at their report (illustrated in Figure 1), *Penis Size Worldwide by Country,* you can see the wide variety of sizes.

Here's a chart of the average penis size by country, from this report.

Table 1: Average Penis Size by Country[15]

Country:	Avg. Size:	Country:	Avg. Size:	Country:	Avg. Size:
Australia	*5.2" (13.3 cm)*	Brazil	6.2" (16.1 cm)	*Canada*	*5.5" (13.9 cm)*
China	*4.3" (10.9 cm)*	Congo	7.1" (17.9 cm)	*Egypt*	*6.2" (15.7 cm)*
France	*6.3" (16.0 cm)*	India	4" (10.2 cm)	*Japan*	*4.3" (10.9 cm)*
Mexico	*6.2" (15.9 cm)*	Russia	5.2" (13.3 cm)	*Sweden*	*5.8" (14.8 cm)*
UK	*5.5" (13.9 cm)*	USA	5.1" (12.9 cm)	*Venezuela*	*6.7" (17.0 cm)*

Figure 6: World Map of Average Penis Size by Country [14]

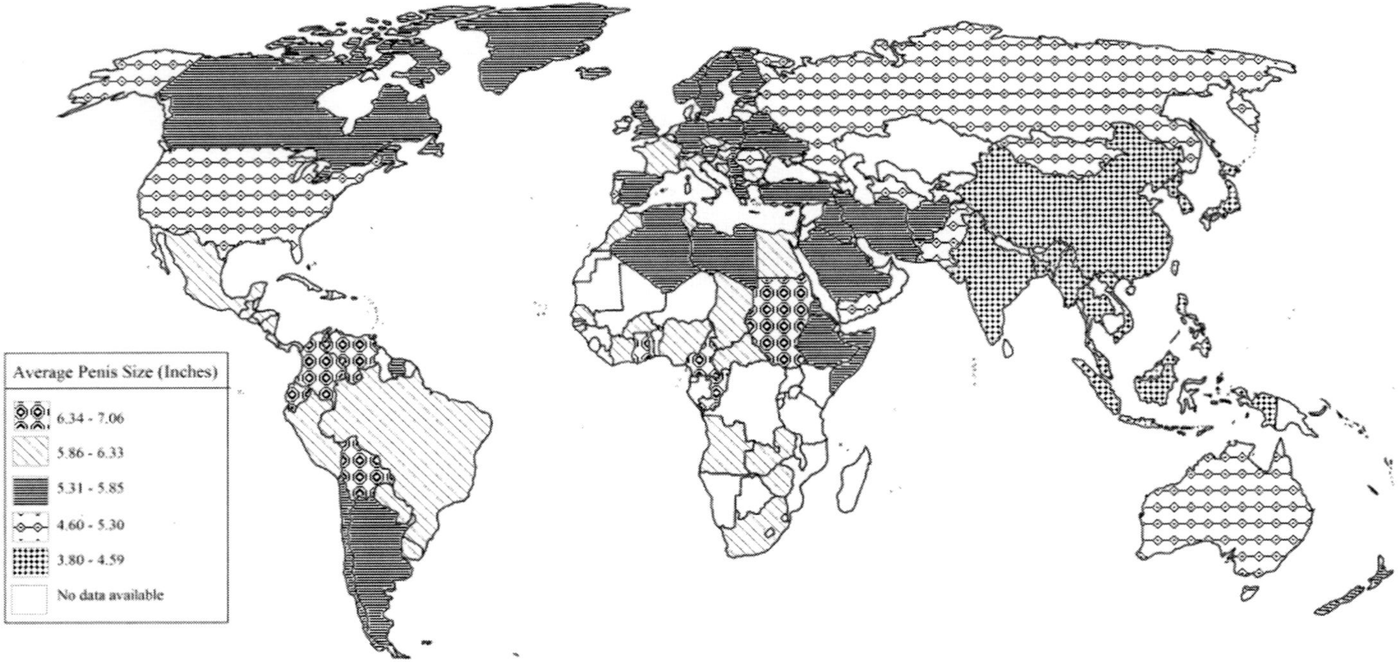

How to Measure Your Penis

If you're still concerned about your size, following are instructions on how to properly measure your penis. To measure the length:

- Stand up.

- Bring yourself to a full erection and, hold your penis parallel to the floor.

- Locate the pubis by pressing a finger against your body at the top part of the shaft where it joins your abdomen.

- Measure from the pubis to the tip of the glans. Use a plastic ruler to allow you to press one end against the pubis and lay the ruler flat along the penis. This enables you to read off the length.

To measure the girth, it doesn't really matter where you take this measurement, as long as for comparative purposes you always do it at the same point. Girth is generally taken at a point mid-way along the shaft while erect. A tailor's cloth measuring tape is ideal, but a piece of string wrapped around the girth and held where the end of the string meets itself will work. Then place the string alongside a ruler and this will give you the circumference (girth).

Losing Weight and Penis Length

One of the easiest ways to increase penis length is to lose weight. Although this doesn't really lengthen the penis, it does increase the "usable" length of the penis. There is a *suprapubic* fat pad located right above the penis. With weight gain, like other fatty areas of the body, this fat pad grows thicker, and reduces the exterior length of the penis. For obese men, weight loss not only can have all the health benefits that come with losing weight, but can also result in a significantly longer exterior penis. Even men who just have a few pounds to lose can not only enjoy increased stamina from weight loss, but a longer penis as well.

Premature Ejaculation

Premature ejaculation affects all males at some time, most often during teen years and into the twenties. An estimated one-third of American men aged 18 to 59 are thought to be affected, making the condition twice as common as erectile dysfunction. A senior executive of one of the world's largest condom manufacturers told me the most frequently asked question they receive is, "How can I prevent premature ejaculation?"

It's been theorized man was designed to ejaculate quickly in order to keep copulating time to a minimum—just as it is in the animal world. In this way, they would avoid becoming an easy target for predators. Evolution hasn't changed this protective response, and man has to learn how to overcome this biological tendency to cum quickly, to bring greater enjoyment to both him and his partner.

Avoid Disappointment

Over time, and with the growing familiarity of a lifetime partner, the confidence gained will help a man avoid the disappointment that usually accompanies premature ejaculation. Indeed, when men pass their mid-fifties, the reverse will most likely be true. One of my old friends described how much better sex was for him and his partner now they had reached middle-age. He enjoyed it so much, he never wanted to stop. His wife would taunt him with the question, "Aren't you ever going to cum?"

There are creams men can buy and apply to the penis. These deaden the sensory nerves so reaching a climax becomes more of an effort. This, in my opinion, is not a good idea. First, it isn't going to train men in penis control, so when the cream is not applied the problem remains. Second, there is a risk of applying some of the cream inside the woman's vagina as the penis rubs along her sensory walls, and that is something you definitely don't want to do!

Be In Control

Guys, if you want to last longer and be in control of the point of no return (PONR), you need to practice self-control. Here's an exercise to help your body learn how to beat the premature urge every time you make love. This exercise is best performed in private and on your own at first. Here's the routine:

Edging

Edging is fairly easy and can be extremely effective.

1. Lie back and bring yourself as close to the PONR as you dare.

2. Immediately stop all movement.

3. Take a deep breath and clamp the base of your penis between your finger and thumb tightly to prevent fluid flow.

If you fail to prevent ejaculation this first time, it's not unusual. Try again after an hour or so (or even another day). However, this time stop sooner. Instead of clamping off between your finger and thumb, you can also apply pressure at the *frenulum* immediately below the head (glans) of the penis. Try both ways.

Remember, we're all different. Your control may be greater or lesser than others. Try this exercise with and without clamping off. Stick with what suits you best. Edge closer to ejaculation each time, and you will discover just how close you can get to it without actually cumming.

When you have successfully edged to the closest point of ejaculation the first time, relax and let your erection subside. Stimulate again as close as you dare to the point of no return, stop all movement and breathe deeply while clamping off. Then relax for 30 seconds, before repeating the whole routine. Repeat this exercise four times.

By now, you will be getting the idea and gaining confidence—you may even wish to go on to completion as a reward to yourself. In addition to avoiding premature ejaculation, if you don't go on to ejaculate, but instead save it for an hour or so before orgasm, you will notice an increase in semen volume. There can be variations in timing and volume from one man to another, but it may be something you'd like to experiment with.

Replicate the Exercise

When making love you can't replicate this exercise in quite the same way. Be patient. You may still need some practice to control your ejaculation, but the initial exercises will have helped you learn how far you can take it before going over the edge. Remember, there is a big difference between self-stimulation and penetration. Sensitivity and the sensual thrill increases substantially during penetration—all the more reason for effective control.

Having practiced the routine described, and when making love with your partner, you should withdraw and keep perfectly still while breathing deeply and clamping off your penis when you get close to climax. Allow a little time to regain control, and then you can penetrate again. Don't be surprised if you swiftly arrive at the PONR once more. If this happens, give yourself more time to relax and allow the urge to ejaculate to subside.

Share what you are doing with your partner—she will know how to help by keeping still at the right moment. She will recognize the need, because she can do precisely the same for herself if arriving close to her own PONR and wishing to extend the lovemaking. There will come a time when both of you will be able to control the urge to climax and decide for yourselves when you want to orgasm just by slowing the rhythm and picking up speed again when you're ready. Climaxing together can be very satisfying.

Continued Practice Brings Results

The more frequently you practice edging, the quicker you will be able to control the timing of your ejaculation. Here's a tip: when you get close to ejaculation, take a deep breath and think about something really mundane—like raking the backyard or whatever you consider to be the least sexy thing you can imagine.

Progress Gradually

As you grow more confident, you will be able to have penetrative sex and, instead of withdrawing at the crucial moment, simply stop thrusting and take a deep breath. If your partner recognizes the sudden intake of breath as the signal to stop moving, they can also help. Continue thrusting well after the feeling of ejaculation subsides. That's important.

You don't have to just lie there frozen still. Don't forget you still have lips to kiss and hands to caress. If your partner would prefer you to ejaculate at that point, she won't stop her movements—and you'll both be happy!

Another Way

NOTE: You've got to be fit to do this one!

I don't have to tell you your erection subsides as soon as you have ejaculated, but imagine what it would be like to enjoy the spasms of orgasm without ejaculating, so your penis stays hard and erect and ready to orgasm again. With a really fit *pubococcygeus* (PC) muscle, you can squeeze it so hard it traps the seminal fluid and, even though the orgasmic contractions occur, the seminal fluid is retained—and so is your erection!

In Chapter 7—The Love Muscle, I'll show you how to get your PC fit. Premature ejaculations will not only be a thing of the past, you can also become a multi-orgasmic man!

Proof That It Works

A married 35-year-old student of lovemaking techniques contacted me, seeking help with mild and sporadic erectile dysfunction. I told him about the PC muscle and gave him a simple routine to get it really fit, just as described in Chapter 7: The Love Muscle. Here's what he said:

> *I've been getting some solid results thus far. My erection quality is through the roof, but what is really exciting is that by doing those 30 second Kegel holds, then release for 5 seconds, has taken me to another level in the bedroom. I can now actually partially ejaculate (since I do a Kegel squeeze when I'm close to the PONR) and it stays hard like nothing happened. WOW!! I'd only done that 1 or 2 times in my teens and early 20s. Over the past week, I've done that 7 times.*

Erection Quality (EQ)

EQ is an abbreviation used to describe the overall performance of an erect penis, its degree of hardness and its staying power. One of the greatest concerns for a man is when he is unable to achieve a full and hard erection, he sporadically loses the ability to get an erection at all or his erections subside unexpectedly. Nothing else makes him more despondent or depressed and kills his confidence. This is described as Erectile Dysfunction (ED) and sometimes as impotence.

The word 'impotence' conjures up images, especially to the sufferer, of a man who has nothing to offer the world. He cannot father a child, and he is missing the very essence of manhood. Let me dispel this myth straightaway.

You are no less of a man if you have any of the variations of ED. You can still produce sperm and, in the hands of a caring, understanding and loving partner, you can still be brought to orgasm with only a partial erection!

Erectile Dysfunction

Did you know ED can strike at any age? It occurs from as young as 20 and with increasing probability as you get older. The causes are varied, but usually it's either physical (70%) or psychological (30%). ED can also be caused by hormonal deficiencies, stress or even guilt!

Good Tubes

Great erections are all based on great circulation. The blood vessels supplying the penis are not as big as you might think. Compared with some other blood vessels in the body, they're quite small—only 2 to 3mm in diameter. They may be small, but they are flexible. The smooth muscle of these tiny tubes contain within their walls an enzyme called nitric oxide synthetase. When triggered by a rush of nitric oxide, typically through sexual stimulation, these vessels expand allowing more blood to flow into the spongy tissues of the penis than flow out. Result—an erect penis.

Don't Ignore The Symptoms

If the blood vessels are restricted, a successful erection becomes more difficult. There are a number of reasons this may happen and investigations by a medical practitioner, or referral to a urologist, might be indicated.

You may have heard of 'hardening of the arteries' as we age. When this happens, the arteries become narrow and less flexible. This is most often caused by cholesterol deposits building up in vital blood vessels and is described as atherosclerosis. Hardening of the arteries can negatively affect your erection quality.

The symptoms of ED can also indicate the possible onset of diabetes. For this reason, it is important not to ignore ED and hope it goes away. Talk to a doctor. He will take into account all the other facets of your lifestyle and help you arrive at an accurate diagnosis with sensible actions to take in order to avoid any serious illness and to get your penis performing again.

Get Checked Out

With a simple blood test, a doctor can check your levels of testosterone, a much needed hormone to maintain the levels of nitric oxide synthetase in your penis. Your doctor will probably check out your fundamental systems—heart and nervous system—and consider your physical fitness. Weight loss (where indicated) and increased physical activity improve erectile function in about one-third of patients.

For those already taking medication for another ailment, it could be the medication itself suppressing the body's production of nitric oxide, and now we know what that means! No increased blood flow— no erection! There is a growing belief that NSAIDs (non-steroidal anti-inflammatory drugs) can also have this effect. Additionally, it has been established some medications for blood pressure and cholesterol may also have erectile dysfunction as a side effect.

Alternate Treatments for ED

After you have been checked out by your doctor and everything is okay, what should you do if your EQ still isn't as good as you'd like? After talking to your doctor about your plans, you may consider one of these alternatives:

Supplements:

- Sildenafil (Viagra), tadalafil and vardenafil work by increasing nitric oxide levels.

- Testosterone patches or gel: If your testosterone levels are low, this may be prescribed. The gel is rubbed on the skin a few times a week or possibly daily. Use this per the advice of your physician following your check-up.

Injections:

- Using a micro needle, alprostadil or papaverine is injected directly into the penis.

- Pellet of alprostadil can also be inserted into the urethra using a specially designed inserter.

Cock Ring:

- A cock ring is a latex ring mounted around the base of the penis. It partially restricts blood flow out of the penis to improve erection quality.

Penis Pump:

- A penis pump is a clear tube fitted over the penis and connected to a mechanical pump that extracts air from inside the tube. This encourages blood to flow into the penis due to the reduced pressure. Erection is maintained by a rubber ring fitted to the base of the penis.

Pros and Cons of Alternative Treatments

Spontaneity is something we all love about the sudden rush of lust that leads to immediate uninhibited sex. Unfortunately, most of those alternative treatments listed above require some planning, if not actual application, and spontaneity is lost. Nonetheless, it's worth noting a few things about some of them.

Sildenafil (Viagra):

Please know, if you do not have erectile dysfunction, taking this drug will not make any difference to your erections. In fact, regularly and frequently taking this drug, when it is not necessary, can lead to you becoming dependent on it.

With sildenafil, you will not have an erection unless you are sexually stimulated. Although sildenafil can increase blood flow to the same genital areas as a man, administering this drug to women will not have the same effect. Sildenafil does not increase a woman's desire.

Sildenafil can be purchased in various sized tablets. Unless you need the strongest size (100mg), always take only the amount required to achieve a full erection.

TIP: The 50mg size suits many men, and the cheapest way to buy these is to purchase the 100mg tablets and cut them in half.

The time taken for sildenafil to take effect varies from man to man, but can range from 15 to 60 minutes. Generally speaking, the heavier the man, the longer it takes. This drug stays effective for up to four hours. This is not to say you can stay hard for four hours. It means it will meet sexual stimulation with an erection for up to four hours after you take the tablet.

Tadalafil (Cialis):

Tadalafil is a PDE5 inhibitor that produces the same result as sildenafil but is taken in a lower dose—20mg. It is worth trying as an alternative to sildenafil, because although more expensive than sildenafil, it extends the period of usefulness after taking the tablet to as much as 36 hours or even longer. There is a growing belief in the efficacy of a daily, low-dose (2.5 mg) of Cialis in certain cases. Discuss this with your doctor.

Testosterone:

Don't play around with testosterone unless under the supervision of your medical practitioner. It is a powerful hormone that influences much more than just your sex drive. However, don't forget plenty of exercise keeps your levels topped up at their peak.

Injections and Pellets:

I have yet to hear from anyone who has persevered with these. I understand the results can be long lasting and even painfully hard erections. Here again, discuss this with your doctor before giving this alternative treatment a try.

Cock Rings:

Cock rings can be effective, especially in the early stages of ED where an erection is attainable but subsides early. They are available in many sizes and many materials. Avoid the metal rings; these can be dangerous if fitted so tight you cannot remove it—a visit to the hospital is embarrassing at best. Latex is good. Try the smaller rings designed to go around the base of the penis and the slightly larger that allow the complete set of genitalia to be restricted, by including the testicles. This latter idea also increases the sensitivity of penis and testes for the man by restricting blood flow away from the genitalia and tightening the scrotum. Choose a cock ring that incorporates a clit-tickler for sharing the benefits of wearing a ring with your partner when grinding pelvises together.

Penis Pumps:

The penis pump is another device, which takes time and can cause spontaneity to disappear. The cylinders come in different sizes, so choose one that is right for you. The best ones are made from thick and solid acrylic and differing sizes are supplied to order. The manufacturers tell you how to size-up. Resist the temptation to lie—it makes no difference to them how big or small you are. It's important the cylinder is right for your size.

In addition to the tube, a penis pump also has a pump to create a vacuum within the cylinder. Many have just a rubber squeeze-ball to pump out the air. Some come with an electrically-driven pump. The best are those with a trigger-style pump with a vacuum gauge, so you know how much pressure is being applied.

Never pump too hard; you might burst a blood vessel! -6 Hg or -0.2 Bar is plenty of vacuum pressure and allows the blood to engorge your penis gently. Remove the cylinder, leaving the rubber ring around the base of your penis and, hey presto!, you have an erection.

IMPORTANT: Don't leave the erection-retaining rubber ring in place for more than 30 minutes; you could injure yourself—not only embarrassing at the hospital but painful, too!

Harder Erections, Increased Girth and Greater Ejaculations

Here is a natural way to improve your EQ—no pills or potions or gadgets required. All you'll need is your hands.

1. Stroke to a full erection, but not beyond the PONR—in other words don't cum.

2. When fully erect, stop stroking but simply gently rub anywhere along the shaft that will keep the erection at its peak without spilling over to an orgasm.

3. Continuing this exercise for 20 minutes.

This is also described as ballooning because, over time (3 months and more, when carried out at least 5 times a week) you will see an increase in penis girth, as well as a greater hardness to your erections. If you avoid ejaculating completely for three or four days while exercising like this, you will notice an increase in the volume of ejaculate, which provides a much stronger kick to your orgasms.

Penis Enlargement (PE)

Much has been written about penis enlargement, and there's quite an industry out there taking advantage of men who think their favorite member is too small. First, having read this far you should have received the message—a large penis is NOT the most important thing in a woman's life. Second, you really do have only two choices if you want a bigger penis: surgery or exercises.

Surgery is expensive and not without risk. Additionally, it is not always successful. Pills and supplements won't do it—despite all the claims you may have read. The more honest of those pushing the pills give you exercise routines to use while taking the supplements. Hanging weights does work but can be dangerous, unless done under specialist supervision. Penis pumps provide a temporary increase but often distort the shape if not used properly.

Having studied this subject over many years and written a book about penis enlargement, I can vouch for the fact that penis enlargement using your hands only does work. However, you have to be patient, dedicated to the program and believe in what you're doing. This is not an instant solution. Many students of PE have taken years to achieve their goals.

How PE Exercises Make Your Penis Grow

When you exercise your body, you stretch tissues and ligaments, and your blood circulation increases. Circulation is the key to a successful workout; blood removes carbon dioxide from the exercised tissues and expels it through the lungs. The lungs take in fresh oxygen, which the blood transports back to the worked areas. The blood not only brings in oxygen but also the nutrients needed for the production of new cells. This, albeit very basic explanation, is how bodybuilders achieve their results.

If penis enlargement is so different from body building, how can it be achieved even though it is not a muscle? As the penis doesn't have muscles (only smooth muscle) to work out, you have to provide that missing link—with your hands!

Doesn't having an erection provide that stretch? **No.**

Not even by masturbation? **No, again.**

Think about it. If your penis stretched more every time you had an erection, how big do you think it would be today?!

Avulsions:

Body tissue stretched just a little bit more than its natural elasticity will create avulsions. An avulsion is a microscopic tear. At the cellular level, it means the body will call up the necessary building blocks to create new cells at the point of the tear. As I said before, these building blocks are delivered by the blood. Continue the exercises on a regular basis and the new cells create not only flesh but blood vessels and all the other tissues essential for a working torso. So far, it is no different to the bodybuilder.

Now you understand why through stretching new cells are grown, and this makes it possible to target a specific area and expect to see it grow. It is important you reach an understanding of what you are considering doing, which is why I recommend you study the subject, as written by experienced practitioners, and join a recommended online forum. In an online forum you can, with complete anonymity, seek advice and help and join in the fraternity that has built up around this subject over the years.

The Early Boner

How man has physically evolved over the millennia is amazing. Before we began to walk upright, man had a penile bone, like all other mammals.

Evolution has changed that. Human mammals are now the only mammalian species without a penile bone. It is thought when our ancestors began to walk upright, the penis was exposed, risking damage, so man evolved a boneless penis to protect it.

Spikes

Early man also had spikes on his penis to remove the sperm of others who had mated with a female, much like a cat. The purpose of these spikes were to ensure his semen would be implanted instead of the previous male's. Thankfully, as we evolved to become monogamous, the spikes disappeared. The coronal rim around the base of the head is all that is left of that inherited shape.

Monogamy

Research, by Dr Susanne Schultz and colleagues from the University of Manchester, England, suggests humans became monogamous to protect their children from being killed by other males. Infants were most vulnerable while still dependent on their mothers, who would delay further conception while nursing their young. This, in turn, meant that killing children encouraged mating sooner for the male[16]. As monogamy began to emerge, males were more likely to share in child care, which may also to have led to the development of more complex brains.

The Seven Year Itch

It seems like the "Seven Year Itch" has been extended nowadays. A survey of 3,000 married people, carried out by an online dating agency, showed that they began to get bored with their spouse after ten years and eleven months. The survey suggests that after a decade of marriage the romance often dies and partners have become disillusioned with their routine life.

- 25 percent said their marriage had lost its sparkle, because they no longer bother to go out together or make romantic gestures.

- 20 percent said their sex life had reached the point where they no longer got excited at the thought of making love.

- 12 percent could not remember the last time their partner paid them any sort of compliment.

A spokesman for the dating site that carried out the survey said, "It takes a special someone to step back from everyday life and realize it takes a bit of effort to keep the romance alive. And the fact our couples mentioned their sex life not once, but three times in the top ten list indicates this is one area which falls by the wayside after several years of marriage."[17]

Further Reading

- *Penis Exercises: A Healthy Book for Enlargement, Enhancement, Hardness, & Health*—by Rob Michaels

- *How to Maximize Your Manhood: What Every Red-Blooded Male Needs to Know*—by Clive Peters

- Online Penis Enlargement Forum: http://www.PEGym.com (Free to Join)

- Online Penis Enlargement Forum: http://www.Thundersplace. com (Free to Join)

——— 5 ———

Breasts

B is for breasts,
Of which ladies have two;
Once prized for the function,
Now for the view.

~ Robert Paul Smith

When I began researching material to relate all things sexual and about the relationships between the sexes, I began to list anatomical parts that most often come into play. "Breasts" were at the bottom of the list and were followed by a question mark.

Are breasts sexual organs?

What is it about breasts that attract and intrigue us so much? Why is this not true in some parts of the world? The primary function of breasts, after all, is to feed the a woman's child until it is old enough to no longer be dependent on their mother's body for food.

"Oh, come on!" my male friends exclaim in disbelief. "How many men do you know who don't find a nice pair of tits attractive? Haven't you ever spotted nice cleavage that suggests a full and firm bosom lies hidden beneath? Why are there so many men's magazines that feature pictures of topless women. Why do women worry so much about the size and shape of their own breasts?"

If we are going to understand what it is about breasts that intrigue us—and that applies to both sexes—these questions, and many more, can't be ignored.

The Rooting Instinct

We, and by "we" I mean both sexes, are introduced to the usefulness of breasts, and nipples especially, at a very early age. Nursing or suckling babies are born with a rooting instinct to bring their mouth toward whatever is touching their face. For this reason, lips and mouth taking in a nipple and the surrounding area (*areola*) comes naturally to everyone.

However, that's not going to induce sexual arousal, is it? Maybe not, but it is going to get the chemistry going—and here's where suckling can lead to sexual arousal.

Breasts and Sexual Arousal

In Chapter 8: The Chemistry of Love and Lust, we will talk more about what the brain and body does to bring couples together. However, when it comes to breasts, it's the cuddle hormone, oxytocin, flooding the body when there is naked touching, that enhances sexual arousal. Feeling skin—to-skin contact of the female's breasts brings to life a set of pleasure hormones. These opioids are morphine-like chemicals that come into to play to reduce pain awareness and create feelings of elation.

"Coming into play" is an apt description at this point. The combination of elation and reduced sensitivity to pain allows the female to enjoy playful activities employing her breasts, which she might not ordinarily even consider. Each to their own preferences, of course, and it must be remembered what one will enjoy, another may abhor.

Erotic Receptors

Both sexes have nipples, but female nipples are more sensitive due to the increased number of nerves and nerve endings.[18] A female's nipple sensitivity will vary during her menstrual cycle, but during arousal they generally become stiff, erect and protrude out. The size and protrusion varies from woman-to-woman, as does the area and pigmentation of the surrounding areola.

The nipples and areolas of both males and females can be erotic receptors. Sometimes the sensation is intense enough to bring about an orgasm in individuals of either sex.

Breasts and Sexual Play

There are numerous ways breasts come into sexual play. Examples can include:

1. Gently biting,

2. Pinching,

3. Rolling of nipples between finger and thumb, or even

4. Ejaculating directly onto the nipples and surrounding areas.

Larger Breasts Wrapped Around a Man's Penis

Women with larger breasts can wrap their breasts around a man's penis as a form of sexual play. The female lies on her back, and the male straddles her chest. He thrusts his penis back and forth between her breasts. She can add to the pleasure by holding a breast in each hand and squeezing them together around his penis.

Her pleasure comes from the friction of his penis and testicles riding her breasts. His pleasure comes from both the physical activity and the clear view of what is happening. Lubrication adds greatly to the sensation.

If the male wishes to climax using this method, the female can either look down on his penis head and open her mouth, to take his ejaculate or guide his penis with her hands so it splashes over her breasts. Use this as a prelude to vaginal penetration or vice-versa. Make your own rules!

Sexual Organs

All of this begs the question: Are breasts sexual organs?

Here's an extract from views published on the Internet, ending with an amusing anecdote by author Carolyn Latteier, the author of *Breasts, The Women's Perspective on an American Obsession*, in a TV program "All About Breasts":

> *Certainly people in the US, UK, Australia, and other countries think of breasts as being a sexual organ. However, the obvious biological function of breast is to make milk for the baby.*
>
> *Human reproduction can certainly be carried on without ever touching the breasts, so breasts are NOT inherently a sexual organ.*
>
> *But are they somehow both a feeding machine and secondarily a sexual organ, as many think? Consider the fact that about 100 years ago woman's ankles were very sexual in men's minds. And tiny feet were a fetish for Chinese men in times past. All kinds of parts of female body have been inspiring to men during history and in various cultures, so we ask you to consider that breasts simply have been turned into a similar fetish in US society and others influenced by it.*

Breasts are a part of the "whole package of a woman", and men can easily respond sexually to seeing a woman—but the difference is that breasts in themselves are not any special "arousal" machines or obsession points UNLESS the influences from around you have wired your brain to think so. In other words, if a man grows up without this "BREASTS = SEX" influence from media, TV, magazines, and peers, then to him, female breasts will not be any more special than a woman's face, feminine hair, wide hips, narrow waist, or other such feminine characteristics.

Well, we do have a peculiar obsession with breasts in this culture. A lot of people think it's just the human nature to be fascinated with breasts but in many cultures, breasts aren't sexual at all. I interviewed a young anthropologist working with women in Mali, in a country in Africa where women go around with bare breasts. They're always feeding their babies. And when she told them that in our culture men are fascinated with breasts there was an instant of shock. The women burst out laughing. They laughed so hard, they fell on the floor. They said, "You mean, men act like babies?"[19]

Breast Comparisons

There are as many women unhappy with the size and shape of their breasts as there are men who are equally unhappy with their genitalia. Both sexes go to the Internet to see what 'normal' sizes and shapes look like—for reassurance or to see what surgical augmentation might do for them.

In the interest of research, I posted a blog headed 'Big Penis Pictures' and guess what happened? Hits on my blog more than tripled!

Recognizing this might be construed as a tease, I wrote my blog visitors might be disappointed to discover there aren't any pictures of big penises on my website, but I provided a website URL that would take them to such pictures.

The problem here, for both sexes, is pictures and videos of breasts and penises abound online, but the most perfect shapes and sizes are always featured. This is further depressing those who think they are, somehow, below what is an attractive or even normal look. Browsing the internet, I came across an excellent website that featured non-sexualized photos of normal breasts.

Part of the reason why women are unhappy with their breasts is due to the media. From momentarily topless starlets in movies to full—blown porn stars, the media has purported the ideal of big and perky breasts, with small nipples and areolas. However, in reality, the female breasts come in a variety of shapes and sizes. The website *007 Breasts* features pictures of normal breasts—"big, small, sagging, asymmetrical; big areolas or nipples."[20]

This website not only publishes pictures of normal breasts from contributors to the site, but it also publishes the comments made about them by their owners. They talk about sagging breasts, small breasts, flat chests, breast implants, what most teenage girls worry about, breast development, and a lot more.

Symmetry

The size of a woman's breasts vary over the course of her monthly cycle due to water retention and cell growth. Interestingly, most women's breasts are generally not symmetrical. For the average woman, one breast is nearly one-fifth of a cup size bigger than the other.

Nobody really knows why such asymmetry occurs, although genetics are thought to play a part. Also, going through pregnancy and menopause—both hormonal events—can lead to a change in what were previously more matching breasts. As with a man's left testicle being the one that hangs lower than the right, it is the left breast that is the more common to fill out up to a cup size more than the right.

Augmentation

Styles and fads, promoted by the media, come and go. What is in fashion today, goes out of fashion tomorrow. With surgical augmentation, it is good to remember it may be fashionable for you to go up or down a cup size today, but it may not be fashionable a short time away. Surgery is not a routine to put your body through without serious considerations first.

<u>Why do it?</u>

Major health problems aside, most women are prepared to go under the knife for the same reasons men decide to take the surgical route for penis enlargement. The big (pardon the pun) difference is— although a woman's assets may be hidden under clothing, their size remains apparent to everyone. It's this public display that can affect a woman's self-esteem. In contrast, a man, even though the results are not apparent until he is undressed, might decide on augmentation for different reasons, but the psychological result is the same for both sexes—to feel better about themselves and gain confidence.

Here's what Julia Stephenson has to say about breast augmentation, "I wonder why I put my body through so much upheaval. What made me think that a bigger bosom would make me happier?"[21]

In an extract from Stephenson's book, published in YouMag she went on to say,

> *My boyfriend of six years had held a candle for me for years, since long before my boob job. We got together after I had my implants, but now I've had them removed, he doesn't bat an eyelid. Like many British men, he is a bottom and leg man anyway. American men seem more interested in enormous boobs, but that's their problem. Men are not nearly so concerned by our seeming imperfections as we think.*[22]

As the writer, Julie Birchill, puts it, "Men couldn't care less—they generally want women to have a wash, bring beer, show up, and strip off."[23]

Julia Stephenson added, "We mustn't mutilate ourselves because of media pressure, glossy magazines and TV story lines such as those on *Desperate Housewives* where Lynette pulls off a huge business deal because men are mesmerized by her pregnancy-inflated breasts."[24]

One Woman's View

Here's what writer and editor, Kimberly Wylie, has to say on the subject of breast augmentation.

There is a valid point in wanting to feel comfortable in your own skin. As a woman, I want to look good. I want people to find me physically attractive. Our breasts are on display—clothes on or off. It's not surprising so many women are concerned with how theirs look.

If you are so unhappy with what God/nature/genetics (whichever you believe) gave you, or with what the ravages of time or children have taken away from you, your self confidence suffers. Breast augmentation may be an option for you. However, it should only be done because you really want it, not because of your partner's desires.

Surgery, obviously, can have serious complications. As such, having your boobs done shouldn't be taken lightly. However, just as we dye our hair, shave our legs, put make-up on, wear designer duds, and head to the gym to tone our tummies, humans are superficial creatures. Right or wrong, society does judge us by our looks, and if a woman is so unhappy with her breasts that it negatively affects her self-esteem, I don't think anyone should begrudge her enhancing her breasts.

One Man's View

As a man, all I can add is natural breasts do have a unique, soft, sexy feel to them, and, despite being a Brit, I do find a suggestive cleavage a head-turner. However, would I choose one girl over another because she had bigger breasts? No.

For me, the eyes come first, followed by all those other devices we are blessed with: attitude (both physical and mental), ability to communicate (both vocally and subtly), and only then do I notice her hair, her skin, her touch, her perfume, and her warmth.

I'm told half of all women hate their naked body. If you are one of them, please be reassured by the time he sees you naked, he will have already fallen for your other many assets—most of which you won't have even thought about!

Enjoy the love.

6

Hair? Everywhere!

I'm not a finicky person when it comes to pubic hair
maintenance and I certainly don't expect men to shave it all
off, leaving themselves to look like a hairless cat. That's even
creepier than seeing what Austin had, which could really
only be compared to one thing: A clown in a leg lock.

~ Chelsea Handler

It's true, we have hair everywhere! Well, almost. We don't have hair on our lips the palms of our hands or the soles of our feet.

The most obvious place where we have hair is on our head. We cut it, shape it, dye it, grow it long or short, and, above all, wash it frequently. It has been said a head of luxurious hair is a woman's 'crowning glory,' and who would disagree? A head of hair can attract, distract, feel good, and awaken desire.

Body Hair

Some of us have little body hair; some have an abundance. The more obvious body hair locations are under the arms and pubic hair, but we do all have finer hairs covering our entire bodies. Depending mostly on your inherited traits, the color of your hair can vary from the deepest black to the lightest blonde. The density of hair also varies with color. Blondes have between 30 and 50 percent more hair follicles per square inch as a dark-haired person. "Since blonde hair has less pigmentation (fewer melanin molecules) the hair shafts tend to be slimmer, and require more hairs to adequately cover the scalp."[25]

Not every person has under-arm or pubic hair that color-matches the hair on their head. For this reason, it does you no good to guess a beautiful blonde-haired woman has blonde pubic hair. It is usually darker, and sometimes it's the other way around!

Not all Good News

There is one thing we all have in common though—we all sweat!

I was taught it was more polite to describe the topic of sweating as 'horses sweat, men perspire and ladies glow.' Although this may be the more gentlemanly way of addressing this natural process for temperature regulation in the body, there's no getting away from the fact sweaty hair can be pretty unpleasant.

We sweat to take heat away from our body and keep us cool. Hairs are used to wick-away the sweat by evaporation and keep the body at a constant temperature. Body temperature is controlled by the hypothalamus, a heat-sensitive area at the base of the brain. This triggers sweating on the face, neck, chest, and back, as well as from glands across the body called *eccrine glands*.

The characteristic sweat odor, which we often find objectionable, is produced by the glands in the armpits and the groin. These are called the *apocrine glands*. The sweat from these glands is high in a particular protein that is digested by bacteria on the skin. This process produces body odor.

Why We Are Hairy

As I've just explained, hair helps to keep our body temperature stable, but it is also there to protect us. In a small study of volunteers, half of whom had one arm shaved, researchers at Sheffield University, in the UK, found when bed bugs were placed on their skin, the people with shaved arms were bitten more. Sensitive, fine hairs which cover our bodies allow us to feel insects on our skin as well as creating a natural barrier to stop them from biting us, explains study author Professor Michael Siva-Jothy. "The hairs have nerves attached to them and provide us with the ability to detect bugs," he says.[26]

Incidentally, hair is the fastest growing tissue in the body, with bone marrow coming in at a close second.

More or Less Hair

Hair growth is dictated largely by testosterone levels. The most obvious example is in men. Not all men have hairy chests! The variations are the same for women. Yes, women can have hairy chests, usually in the form of a few hairs located around the areolas. The quantity of hair someone has is not always due to the genes passed on from parents. Hair loss or excessive hair growth can be caused by hormonal imbalances.

A close relative worked for some years in the lingerie department of a women's clothing store. It was her job to help ladies choose a bra that was right for them. During fitting sessions involving many hundreds of women over the time she was there, she could not help noticing the high number of women who had hairy nipples.

Women, understandably, can be very sensitive about excessive hair growth. Especially in areas that aren't covered by clothing, such as around the face. This is not rare. As many as one in ten women in the UK have this problem.

Polycystic ovary syndrome (PCOS) is a hormonal imbalance in which a woman's ovaries produce excessive amounts of the male hormone testosterone. This condition produces small, harmless cysts, in addition to excessive hair growth and, in more severe cases, baldness, erratic periods, weight gain, acne, and fertility problems.

It is important to note this condition should not be confused with polycystic ovaries, which simply describes the appearance of small cysts on the ovaries. Approximately 20 percent of women have this condition, with no effects at all and no problems conceiving.

PCOS can run in families and cause no problems at all, apart from *hirsutism*—more hair on the face and/or body than you would expect to find.

Hair Fetish

There is tremendous media pressure on both men and women nowadays to have smooth bodies. It is no wonder there is such insecurity among women, especially young women, who are insecure about their own bodies and unsure what is expected by their peers and sexual partners—especially with their first sexual encounter. What about the guys? What do they like or prefer? What should they do about their own hairy parts?

Merriam-Webster defines 'fetish' as:

> *an object or bodily part whose real or fantasied presence is psychologically necessary for sexual gratification and that is an object of fixation to the extent that it may interfere with complete sexual expression.*[27]

A keen interest in and an obsession for body hair might be described as a fetish. To avoid being called irrational, let's accept there are men who find female body hair intriguing, interesting, sexually stimulating, and don't mind how much or how little of it there is. There are many women who think and feel the same about their own hair, as well as about men's hair.

In the 17th Century, the craze was for enormous spreads of pubic hair. The abundant look was so admired you could cheat a little and purchase a merkin, or pubic wig!. Don't think that this embellishment is no longer available; they are still used in the film industry today.

After years of waxing and the inability to effectively grow out her pubic hair, Kate Winslet wore a merkin for her award winning role in *The Reader.* Merkins aren't just for women. Both Jake Gyllenhaal and Anne Hathaway wore merkins in *Love and Other Drugs.*[28] Other actors have used them to feel less exposed in nude scenes. It's amazing when you think about it. What looks like a splendid display of their own elegantly coiffed pubes to us, allows the wearer to feel like they're giving nothing away.

In the 19th Century, it was fashionable to collect and carry lovers' pubic hair in lockets. Men even displayed trophy hairs in their hats!

At the Metropolitan Police Black Museum, in London, England, where artifacts connected with crime in the London metropolitan area are kept for historical and training purposes, I was shown an example of someone who made a hobby of collecting pubic hair. Notorious serial killer John Christie (1899-1953) was sentenced to death for murdering his wife. Among his belongings was a little tobacco tin—a pocket-sized tin with a hinged lid smokers who rolled their own cigarettes used in those days. The curator opened this tin to show me the contents. In each of the four corners was a small pile of pubic hair, each pile was a different color. Christie had a true fetish for pubic hair and collected a sample to keep from each of his victims.

What is Normal?

'Normal' is as individual as we are. Remember—we're all different! Normal really is in the eye of the beholder, much like beauty. Although society, in many cultures, today are currently promoting less body hair, there are many people who feel the natural occurrence of body hair is not just beautiful, but also sensual.

Scientist Dr. James Tanner, a British pediatrician, has lent his name to a scale defining the five stages of development of pubic hair growth. From the near invisible down of childhood to full adulthood, whatever your personal opinion, there is an interest in pubic hair.

It is quite normal to love body hair; however, it is just one of those things we don't usually talk about. When someone does and goes public about it, it hits the headlines. A 28-year old woman, Emer O'Toole, who had not shaved, waxed or used depilatory cream on her armpits, legs or arms for 18 months, even appeared on early morning TV in the UK. She flaunted her armpits and declared, "I really like my body hair." Her boyfriend was happy with it saying, "Boys don't care. They have body hair so they know it's not disgusting."[29]

There are cultures that believe you should not remove your body hair. There are also countries where you will find armpit hair more commonplace, although there is a growing trend to be clean-shaven in this particular part of the body.

Another TV channel in the UK showed a video of women stating the case for removal of all body hair. Following that program, I was sent a comment by an anonymous viewer:

> I can safely say I am relieved to hear there are other women out there who are just as insecure about the hair on their bodies, but (the TV program) didn't make me feel any better. It made me feel worse. What all the women were saying and the pressure in the media to be hairless is just ridiculous, and this documentary was a bit one-sided. What about the people with a little fetish for hair? It is a real thing! But people might not know this because of the one-sided argument, plus if I leave it my boyfriend doesn't care.

Sensuous

As mentioned, some people find body hair very sensuous. Views from two male correspondents give another view. The first reminded me about not just the sight of, but also the texture, warmth and smell of body hair. His particular fetish is the fine down that can appear on forearms, base of the spine, on the tummy, and front of the thighs. He loves the sensation when he lightly caresses those parts with his lips. My guess is that his partner also enjoys the warmth of his breath and the sensations transmitted by those fine hairs to her sensory nerves, as he moves across her body this way.

The second man, a declared lover of the *hirsute* (a lover of the coarse hair that covers a woman's pubic region), described his lover's pubic hair extending from the pubic area down her thighs. He just adored the feeling of her hair brushing against the cheeks of his face as he went down on her.

There is no doubt there are many people who love body hair. Type 'hairy women' into a search engine, and you can begin to appreciate the number of folks into hair. It's not just those who love to see it, but those who want to show it off too.

You should not feel pressured into following fashion. Body hair is totally natural and there for good reasons. It is apparent some, of both genders, have preferences one way or another. What is normal is sticking with what you feel comfortable and what your partner enjoys.

Why Remove It?

Removing body hair is not new. The question is—why do we do it?

Body builders do it, so they can oil smooth skin to show off the defining lines of body muscle. Film star Jane Russell allegedly persuaded Howard Hughes to let her shave his hairy back. This story was even parodied in Harold Robbins' story, *The Carpetbaggers*, published in 1961. She shaved Hughes, with an open razor, because she preferred a smooth back to run her nails down.

Removal of armpit hair quickly gained popularity with women, and this practice is widespread, especially with the development of modern deodorants and antiperspirants. This is a very feminine activity but hasn't caught on with most men. A hairy man is considered masculine, so he displays his armpit hair.

Clearly, the common societal thinking is underarm hair on a woman is unattractive. Is this because it makes her look more masculine? Conversely, would removal of his armpit hair would make a man appear more feminine?

Body hair also holds body oils, dirt and odors. While some enjoy this, others may find it offensive. We discuss the chemistry behind this in Chapter 8: The Chemistry of Love and Lust.

Influence

With the advent of fast, global communications, especially TV and the Internet, people are exposed to trends they are more likely to follow. Unfortunately, many trends originate from dubious sources.

Take pornography, for instance. Close-up camera work of the most intimate nature requires nothing gets in the way—and this includes hair. The first publicly accessible place, apart from film produced specifically for medical interests, where anyone ever saw a totally denuded body was in pornography. This 'different' idea quickly spread to the more acceptable fashion houses, who demanded their models be perfectly smooth-skinned to display evermore flesh in trendy clothing.

Kids and young adults have no wish to be anything other than trendy, so they enthusiastically seek not only ways to depilate but also how to achieve an attractive and painless result. It's not just the younger generation. Forty-something and beyond females and males are taking up the idea a neat bush is more desirable. As word spreads, even the older generations are paying attention and enjoying a new aspect to their love—lives.

A whole new and growing industry has resulted. Since the 1980s, when waxed bushes started to make an appearance, salons have popped up all around the world. Just one of the London-based salons, with its partner salons overseas, claims to have over a million clients.

The number of people who DIY when it comes to personal grooming add to this number substantially. Although waxing is best carried out by an experienced esthetician in an established salon, depilatory creams and gels and good, old-fashioned shaving can be exercised in the privacy of your own home.

How to Begin

Before you begin the hair removal process, first, ask yourself why you want to change what nature gave you. The answer to this question will help you decide how far you want to go—and where to go.

You might consider seeking guidance from a salon. They will have illustrated brochures to help you choose your preferred pubic coif.

Is your wish to simply avoid that bush-spilling-out appearance when you go down to the beach? Or is it a desire to change from the natural diamond shape to something different?

Photos of what others have done can help you avoid a style that may not be right for you. If you will be waxing, take a mild pain killer to reduce the tears-coming-to-your eyes effect, as the hairs are ripped out.

Remember—fashions come and go. The Brazilian—leaving you with just a landing-strip of hair—was all the rage at one time. Then came the Hollywood—leaving absolutely nothing, anywhere. Salons have stencils with all kinds of shapes and sizes to guide their depilatory activities. However, consider the reaction you hope for the first time (and every time) you go to bed with your lover before making a decision.

The good news? It is hair, and it will grow back eventually, if you choose a style that isn't quite right for you.

Be Practical

It has been said naked genitals increase sensation. The brushing of a hand, lips or anything else across freshly denuded skin produces more intense reactions than if the surface is protected by hair. Waxing can leave you smooth for months, but shaving will only last a few days. Many people don't find three-day old stubble attractive, so regular maintenance is a must, if you want to stay smooth.

If you are in a long-term relationship, you may want to discuss your personal grooming choice with your partner. The experimental stage, when you try out different styles, can be fun! This exploratory time can bring you closer than ever and open up avenues of sexual delight not previously experienced.

NOTE—Shaving—For Women: Most women prefer to wet shave, while under the shower or in the tub. That's fine. However, the best way to avoid ingrown hairs—leaving nasty spots and troublesome rashes—is to brush the hairs BEFORE stepping under the shower. This is particularly helpful when shaving nipple hair, an issue more common in women than some may think.[30]

Manscaping

Personal grooming is not just a female thing. Guys, consider your partner and what they would like. You don't want to go all artistic, then have your girlfriend fall over laughing just at the moment you appear from the shower with a ready-to-go hard on.

Be practical and think of her. When she goes down on you, she doesn't want to be flossing her teeth with your pubic hair. At the least, trim back your bush! You can use scissors (carefully) or a beard trimmer set at medium, to produce a really neat and practical appearance. Asking our female friends for some more practical suggestions, the best advice came from Annie who suggested men should shave their 'lickable parts.' Spelling it out, this means shave your penis shaft down to its root and also your ball sack (scrotum). If you have been hiding your crown jewels behind a luxuriant bush until now, the first thing you and she will notice is your penis looks bigger! Now isn't that something you've always wanted?

—— 7 ——

The Love Muscle

Exercise is done against one's wishes and maintained only because the alternative is worse.

~ George Sheehan

Let's talk about 'the love muscle.'

No, no, young man! Put that away! I'm not talking about your penis!

I'm talking about a group of muscles that without them sex wouldn't be very exciting. Plus, without these muscles, you'd have to be very careful with how you walk or your insides would fall out between your legs!

I'm talking about the *pubococcygeal* (PC) muscle group.

Both men and women have the PC muscle group. It provides the power behind orgasmic contractions for women and keeps the walls of her vagina tight. The fitter a woman's PC muscle, the firmer she can make the opening and the tighter she can grip her lover's penis. This is something you can both benefit from right away! For men, the fitter the PC muscle, the harder the erection and the greater the force behind ejaculation. This is why the PC muscle is often referred to as 'the love muscle.'

This group of muscles form the pelvic floor. You may have heard about the pelvic floor, especially if you or your partner has gone through childbirth. The PC muscle is the muscle that keeps our internal organs just that—internal.

It is slung similar to a hammock, between your legs and from front to back. The urethra, anus and, in the case of women, the vagina all pass through this muscle group. Arnold Kegel, M.D., a gynecologist practicing in the 1940s and 1950s, lent his name to a simple exercise to strengthen this group of muscles. For more than a half a century, this exercise, named after Dr. Kegel, has been taught to women during pregnancy and following childbirth.

Kegels

Here's how to do the Kegel exercise.

1. First, locate and recognize the muscle. Your PC is quite large. Sit on a wooden seat, or any firm surface, wearing nothing or something thin, and flex your PC. You will feel just how large a muscle this is between your legs.

2. Once you've found your PC muscle, when you urinate, squeeze the muscle to stop the flow. You just did a Kegel! Try stopping the flow a couple of times, by flexing and releasing the PC. Once you've mastered this, you're ready to do Kegels without going to the bathroom.

3. Squeeze the PC tight, just as if you were stopping the flow of urine. It's the same action as squeezing your anus tight shut. Hold this for a count of five seconds. Repeat this action ten times for a set of ten Kegels.

4. Practice Kegels every day, The great thing about Kegels is you can do them at any time and anywhere, on an empty bladder. You can start right now! Do ten Kegels while you're

reading this. Simple, isn't it? The first day you can start with ten sets of ten Kegels each.

5. Gradually increase the number of sets you do each day, over the coming weeks. This is an exercise you should make a lifetime habit! A fit PC maintains youthful sexual pleasure at every age, throughout your life.

Remember—we're all different. Just do as many Kegels as you feel comfortable, if the ten sets of ten feel like too much. However, be sure to increase the number of reps you feel your PC will allow, without getting tired.

You can also increase the time you hold each Kegel, along with or instead of increasing the number of reps. You'll know your PC is getting stronger when you can hold the Kegel for longer period of time. A man or a woman who can hold their PC clamped tight for a minute has a really fit group of muscles down there! Don't expect too much too soon though. Work up to it. When your PC muscle is in good shape, you may find you can progress more quickly. The best way to strengthen that love muscle is to get into the habit of exercising your PC every day.

A friend of mine, who spends much of his time driving, told me he does Kegels every time he has to stop at a traffic light. Squeeze your PC every time you sit down for a meal, or every time you think of your partner, or every time the phone rings. Make up your own list of when to Kegel. Just make it a habit. Nobody will ever know you're keeping your love muscle in excellent shape, even if they're sitting right next to you!

Beyond the Kegel

There is another exercise, which is particularly good for women after childbirth. It not only strengthens your PC but also helps you regain a flat tummy!

1. Sit upright on a chair and take a deep breath.

2. Filling your chest with air and pull in your lower tummy muscles, as if you are trying to pull your bottom off the chair.

3. Hold this for a few seconds, release and repeat.

Exercising and Orgasm

There was quite an uproar when a recent study revealed how many women regularly achieve orgasms while exercising. Researchers at Indiana University studied 370 women who had reported having exercise induced orgasm (EIO) or exercise induced sexual pleasure (EISP). Approximately 40 percent of these women had experienced EIO or EISP more than ten times. Many of the women surveyed admitted sex and romance were the last things on their mind. Instead, they found the experience made them self-conscious, and 20 percent reported they could not control the experience. A variety of exercises were found to induce orgasm, including:

- Weight lifting (26.5%)

- Yoga (20%)

- Bicycling (15.8%)

- Running (13.2%), and

- Walking/hiking (9.6%)

These exercises hit the spot centered around the core abdominal muscles—giving the phenomenon the name 'coregasm.' Although the study did not conclude the percentage of women overall who have experienced this type of sexual phenomena while exercising, the study authors note it only took five weeks to recruit the 370 women who had experienced EIO or EISP, which leads them to believe it is not a rare occurrence.[31]

Research leader, Debby Herbenick, explains, "This shows that orgasm is not necessarily a sexual event and may teach us about the bodily processes leading up to women's orgasms."[32]

A final word from Batwoman, "Here's an interesting observation about G-spots. My lover says he thinks mine has increased in size since I started Kegeling regularly." We'll learn more about the G-spot in Chapter 10: The Vaginal Orgasm.

—— 8 ——

The Chemistry of Love & Lust

Love is a matter of chemistry, but sex is a matter of physics.

~Unknown

What attracts us to another person?

Many would answer it's the way a person looks, the way they behave and the way they react to us. However, did you know it is really your brain going through the potential mate selection process? Your brain rejects him/rejects her until it spots a potential partner that fits the basic criteria of 'good for procreation.' When your brain does recognize one of these elusive partners, watch out! It becomes the body's biggest chemical factory, producing hormones that can send you into instant ecstasy and desire.

Back in 1999, in the film, *Notting Hill*—starring Julia Roberts and Hugh Grant—Roberts played an American movie star, and Grant played a bookstore owner. When Grant accidentally spills orange juice on Roberts, he offers his nearby home for her to change, which Roberts accepts. Having only known each other for a few minutes, Roberts surprises Grant by kissing him. This instant attraction—fortunately for Grant's character—was a mutually felt sudden rush of hormones connecting the two with an instant desire for each other.

If this has ever happened to you, lucky you! You probably enjoyed the thrill of feeling the sudden adrenaline rush but held off, for two reasons. First was the fear of offending the other person by just grabbing them and kissing them. Second was the fear of rejection. However, if you felt this instant attraction, chances are you made it a point to see the person again. For most people, if those feelings are still there, they then usually work up the courage to let the other person know they find them attractive and then hope the feelings are mutual.

Lust

Your journey to true love is a complex mix of chemical reactions within your body. These are reactions to what your senses are telling you—sight, smell, touch, taste, and hearing. All you know is you want to be close to this person—to touch, to kiss, to make love.

You can blame the butterflies in your stomach and the urge to copulate on the mixture of dopamine, testosterone and estrogen. Enjoy it while you can; it doesn't last!

This is the stuff of one-night-stands! If you recognize what's going on, but feel it's not right, back off and make a date to meet again some other time. It could be you are actually experiencing initial stages of love, and it just needs time to develop—you wouldn't want to lose 'that loving feeling.' However, it could just simply be lust, and you may want to be more cautious if this is the case.

Attraction

This is the second stage of your journey, when adrenaline, dopamine and serotonin make us incapable of rational thinking. You are in love . . . you think.

You are now in a period of settling down with each other, a period of getting to know each other and realizing your partner is not perfect. You can see flaws in the relationship that irritate you to hell. Depending on how quickly the levels of dopamine and testosterone settle back to normal, this may take some time. Sometimes it takes months or even years. This is when you either stay the course—true love—or end the relationship.

This is the most important stage of your journey together; patience and compassion and respect and intimacy come into play with the help of oxytocin and vasopressin (a receptor for arginine). This creates a bond that should last a lifetime. You have found true love.

Oxytocin is made by the brain during sex, breastfeeding and labor. It is also produced when you're in the company of close friends and people you love or admire. It is often referred to as the 'cuddle hormone.' Although it has a very short half-life, it is a key hormone associated with romantic love and is also vital in forming strong social bonds.

Romantic Love

Psychologist Dr Arthur Aron, a social psychologist at Stony Brook University in Long Island, New York, believes you can generate love simply by sharing intimacies for 30 minutes and then staring deeply into each other's eyes for four minutes. This is my thinking behind making a Lover's Steeple (see more information about this in Chapter 23: Problem Solving).

Dr. Aron said, "If strong feeling is combined with signs they can regulate emotions, to see their partner positively and deal with conflict, then it seems to be really productive in staying with that person."[33]

This was the result of studies of successful relationships with people who had increased electrical activity in the caudate tail, an area of the brain which produces emotional responses to visual beauty. They showed signs of stability, with less activity in the brain area related to addiction, while decreased activity in the medial orbitofrontal cortex, which suggested they were less critical.[34]

Dr. Aron noted, "It does allow us to get at what is really going on inside someone aside from what they tell us."[35] There's no doubt that we can't get away from the fact chemistry is intertwined with our electrical nervous system and fed by signals to the brain by our senses—whether we can sense them or not—and the brain is our 'control room.'

Read about Dr Aron and his students here:

http://www.psychology.stonybrook.edu/aronlab-/

Pheromones

Can chemical signals be odorless? We all know about perfumes. Some perfumes we like better than others. However, we emit our own individual perfumes that don't come with any smell, at least not that we're aware of. These are the odorless pheromones we emit to attract the opposite sex.

If we can't smell them, how do we pick up pheromones? We have a vomeronasal organ, also known as Jacobson's organ, in the nose. This is a chemosensory organ located in the medial wall of the nasal cavity that detects pheromones—the chemical signal that says, "I'm attracted to you, and I want sex."

Endorphins

Endorphins are produced primarily in the pituitary gland but also in the brain and central nervous system. They function as neurotransmitters to interact with receptors in cells located in the parts of the brain responsible for blocking pain and controlling emotions.

You may have heard of people claiming to have had an 'endorphin rush' or even had one yourself. This may have been prompted by exercise, sudden excitement or sex.

There are many different kinds of endorphins, and each can play a part in a different scenario. To give you an idea of just how powerful endorphins can be, beta-endorphins are stronger than morphine, and can play a strong role in sex.

'Not tonight; I've got a headache.'

It's not all bad news for migraine sufferers; they might have a higher sex drive, say American researchers. Sexual desire and migraines have both been linked to the brain chemical serotonin. Too little causes headaches; too much causes low libido.

There could be a self-generated cure here for two types of headaches—migraines and cluster headaches (usually on one side of the head). The theory is sex works by triggering the release of endorphins, the body's natural painkillers, which act on the central nervous system to reduce or eliminate the headache. In a study at the University of Munster, Germany, neurologists collected data on 400 patients who experienced migraines or cluster headaches and who had been treated over a two-year period. They found:

- 33.7 percent had made love while enduring a headache.

Of those, 60.2 percent of migraine patients and:

- 36.7 of men and women with cluster headaches had an improvement in symptoms.

- Men were more likely to benefit than women, with 36.4 percent using sexual activity as a therapy for dealing with their headache.

- 13.7 per cent of women used sex to combat a headache.

- Of the migraine patients who saw an improvement in their pain, 19.2 percent had complete relief from their symptoms,

- 51.6 percent experienced moderate relief, and

- 29 percent reported mild relief.

In total, 42.7 percent of all migraine patients experienced at least 50 percent relief, a response rate as high as in studies of acute medication.[36]

Consultant neurologist Dr Nicolas Silver, of the NHS Walton Centre for Neuroscience and Neurosurgery in Liverpool, England, said, "This is a preliminary study, limiting conclusions that can be reached. We can now say, however, that the excuse of 'not tonight; I have a headache' may not be taken seriously by all sexual partners." Scans have shown that the hypothalamus region of the brain is active during a cluster headache, and the same area shows activity during orgasm.[37]

Immunoglobin A

Your production of immunoglobulin A (immune cells that help fight the common cold and flu) is raised 30 percent if you make love one to two times a week, according to American research. Additionally, people who have sex at least 12 times a month have greater heart variability—a measure of how well the heart responds to little changes, which lowers the risk of heart disease, says a study performed at Wilkes University, in Wilkes-Barre, Pennsylvania.[38]

Semen and Sperm

Seminal fluid is such an obvious result of the male orgasm, but what is it made up of?

Doctors Dawn Harper and Christian Jessen described a man's climax, its constituents and how it all happens, like this:

> *It's normal for men to have three to five erections during the night. Men produce around 4,000 sperm a second, but when we ejaculate only around one percent of the semen contains sperm.*[39]

> *Semen is pumped out of the penis at about 10 mph, by the pubococcygeous muscle, which lies within the pelvic floor muscles. On average, a healthy male produces between 2 and 5 ml of semen when he ejaculates—about a teaspoonful, containing anything between 40-600 million sperm.*[40]

At this point, Dr. Harper interjected, "Interestingly, the adult male wild boar produces half-a-liter of semen every time they ejaculate!"

Dr. Jessen continued,

> *Sperm take 75 days to mature in the testicles. The fluid they are transported in is obviously very important. Only a small drop comes from the testicles (to carry the sperm along the vas deferens from the testes to be mixed in with the products of the other glands involved in the production of seminal fluid).*[41]

> *Most of the fluid is produced by the prostate and other glands during arousal and is mostly water, but there are other constituents of the semen:*

> • *Proteins—that coat the sperm and help them when they enter the vagina.*

> • *Sugars—from which the sperm get their energy.*

- *Antioxidants—that help the fertility of the sperm.*

- *The mineral, Zinc—which stabilizes the DNA and helps protect the genetic information held within the sperm.*

- *And, another mineral, Selenium.*[42]

At the point of ejaculation, the fluid is quite thick and gloopy, but soon afterward it becomes more liquid. This fluid has two roles: First, to provide a liquid to carry the sperm as they swim to reach an egg in the woman's ovaries and, secondly, to protect the sperm from attack by the vagina's natural defenses on their way.[43]

Dr. Jessen concluded with this sensible advice, "If you have any queries about your fertility, there are specialist clinics where you can have your sperm analyzed for numbers and motility."[44]

Faster Moving Sperm

Although we know seminal fluid is ejected at a fast rate, the speed with which individual sperm can swim within this fluid depends on the length of their tails. The longer the tail, the faster it can swim.

Studies from the University of Exeter in the UK have found sperm moves at 10 cm per hour—that's 0.005 mph—one tenth the speed of a snail. At this rate, given the average distance a sperm has to travel, a sperm can reach the female's egg within a half hour.[45]

A University of Copenhagen study found sperm in men with high levels of vitamin D move faster. The vitamin may boost levels of calcium, helping to make sperm more mobile.[46]

I do know that relocating to a warmer climate in the winter months reduces blood pressure, because the blood vessels relax and widen—good for sex—and that exposure to sunshine increases the body's vitamin D, through its own natural processes. Maybe this is one reason why sunshine and sex are often associated.

Sunshine and Sex

Vitamin D boosts fertility in both men and women. It is also key to balancing sex hormones in women and improving sperm count in men, according to researchers[47]. For women, vitamin D helps boost levels of the female sex hormones progesterone and estrogen by 13 percent and 21 percent respectively. This regulates menstrual cycles and makes conception more likely.

For men, vitamin D is essential for the healthy development of each sperm's nucleus. It also increases levels of the male sex hormone, testosterone, improving a man's libido. The vitamin's effect on both male and female sex hormones may explain why conception rates fall in the winter and peak in the summer, in Northern European countries, say the researchers at the Medical University of Graz in Austria. In their own study of nearly 2,300 men, they also found levels of testosterone and vitamin D peaked in August and were lowest in March, just as winter was coming to an end. Women had been found to ovulate less, and their eggs have a reduced chance of implanting in the womb, in the winter months.[48]

Use it or Lose It

The description, position and function of the male prostate are described in Chapter 3: Anatomy 101. However, it goes without saying, maintaining prostate function and keeping it healthy are of paramount importance. The prostate is partly made up of smooth muscle, helping in the ejaculation of seminal fluid when climaxing. The old saying 'Use it or lose it' can be applied to the prostate gland.

Climaxing exercises the prostate muscle. Exercise is good. Ejaculate often and regularly throughout life and keep up the Kegel exercises, and you could be extending your sex life beyond expectations.

Extend Your Life

A study of men aged 45 to 50, in South Wales, UK, (the Caerphilly Cohort Study) found regular sex has a protective effect. Those men who enjoyed frequent orgasms (twice a week) had a fifty percent lower risk of early death than those who missed out.[49]

One American expert estimated sex at least three times a week can add two years to your life, by increasing heart rate and blood flow. Do it every day and your life expectancy could increase by 8 years! Although this is just an estimate, and there have been no conclusive studies to prove this theory, it sure is worth trying!

In addition to boosting circulation and reducing stress, sex releases DHEA (dehydroepiandrosterone), a building block of testosterone, which helps repair and heal tissue. It's also a natural anti-depressant, especially for women. DHEA helps maintain muscle tone and keep your skin looking younger. It has also been described as an anti-aging hormone and triples a woman's chance of conception, a trial at Tel Aviv University, Israel, found.[50]

Women undergoing fertility treatment were also six times more likely to give birth to a healthy baby after taking 75mg a day of DHEA. Dr. Norbert Gleicher, a DHEA expert based at the Center for Human Reproduction in New York, believes it makes egg quality better by improving the ovarian environment.[51]

DHEA can be taken orally and is available without prescription in some countries. However, it is **ALWAYS** best to consult your medical practitioner or pharmacist before taking any supplements. Testosterone is available by prescription and is usually given to women as a cream. Both of these hormones can reach lower levels in women, well before menopause has started. The levels can be checked through blood, urine or saliva testing.

For many, replacement DHEA and other hormones can also improve both sleep and mood, both of which are beneficial to raising libido and the enjoyment of sex. HRT, or hormone replacement therapy, can be considered by women whose levels of estrogen and progesterone need replacement following menopause. Ask your doctor about biodentical hormones, to seek advice as to whether that approach could provide a better solution for your individual menopausal symptoms.

Food for Thought—And for Staying Healthy

The prostate gland looks rather like a walnut. (It's ironic walnuts are also good for your prostate.) We've all heard about prostate cancer, and it's good to have regular testing for early detection. However, it's also important to do whatever possible to keep your prostate healthy to begin with, which means watching what we eat. Here are some frightening statistics:

- Other than skin cancer, prostate cancer is the most common cancer in American men.

- About 238,590 new cases of prostate cancer will be diagnosed, in America alone, in 2013.

- About 29,720 American men will die of prostate cancer in 2013.

- About 1 man in 6 will be diagnosed with prostate cancer during his lifetime[52].

- About 41,000 men are diagnosed with prostate cancer annually, in the UK.

- Approximately 324,000 men are diagnosed with prostate cancer annually, in the EU.

- Globally, nearly 900,000 men are diagnosed with prostate cancer each year[53].

The trouble is most news reports tell us about beating cancer after we've been diagnosed with the disease and the best diets to increase chances of survival. Wouldn't it be better to take up those dietary recommendations to *avoid* getting cancer?

A study found those diagnosed with the disease early had a lower risk of the cancer spreading, if they replaced animal fats found in processed foods with healthy vegetable fats. One serving of oil-based salad dressing a day, equivalent to one tablespoon, was linked with a 29 percent lower risk of potentially lethal prostate cancer and a 13 percent lower chance of dying from *any* cause. The American authors stressed the research involving 4,577 prostate cancer patients had revealed an association with a diet of healthy oils, such as those provided by nuts, gave men with prostate cancer the best chance for survival. In an online paper published by the journal JAMA Internal Medicine, they wrote, "Overall, our findings support counseling men with prostate cancer to follow a heart-healthy diet in which carbohydrate calories are replaced with unsaturated oils and nuts to reduce the risk of all-cause mortality."[54]

Of men with prostate cancer enrolled in the study, approximately 20 percent died from the disease by the eighth year. Another 31 percent died from heart disease, and almost 21 percent died from other cancers. At the time they were recruited, all the men had non-metastatic prostate cancer, meaning the disease had not yet spread.[55]

Information about the patients' dietary habits was collected from questionnaires. Swapping animal fats and carbohydrates for healthy vegetable fats, including olive and canola oil as well as oils from nuts, seeds and avocados, was found to have a significant impact on disease progression and death.[56]

Men who replaced 10 percent of their daily carbohydrate consumption with vegetable fats had a 29 percent lower risk of developing deadly prostate cancer and a 26 percent reduced risk of dying from any cause. The study showed eating an ounce of nuts a day led to an 18 percent lower risk of lethal prostate cancer and an 11 percent lower risk of death.[57]

Dr. Erin Richman, from the University of California at San Francisco, said, "Consumption of healthy oils and nuts increases plasma (blood) antioxidants and reduces insulin and inflammation, which may deter prostate cancer progression."[58]

Food for Sex

A well-fed woman is more easily aroused, say researchers in the US. When female hamsters were injected with leptin, a hormone that makes us feel full, they headed straight to the male hamster. Leptin clears the way for other hormones to be produced, which gives arousal a head start.[59]

On the other hand, "A romantic three-course meal doesn't translate into action in the bedroom," says dietician Helen Bond of the British Dietetic Association. "In fact, you're better off having sex *before* you go to the restaurant. Rich, carbohydrate-heavy meals cause a huge energy slump about two hours later, what's known as postprandial dip. As your body focuses on digesting the food, you'll feel sleepy and hardly in the mood for sex by the time you get home."[60]

Many people find making love in the morning the best. You're both rested and hormones are at their optimum. Try breakfast in bed!

Men who regularly eat foods rich in zinc, such as beef, pecans and pine nuts, increase their sperm count by up to 74 percent. Honey boosts libido; it's rich in B vitamins, needed for testosterone production, and its fructose content aids stamina. In ancient Babylon, the bride's father gave his new son-in-law honey beer every day for a month after they married, to put them in the mood for love—which is where we get the term the 'honeymoon.'[61]

Alcohol and Sex

Alcohol releases tension and relaxes you, without reducing desire. However, imbibe too much and sexual performance suffers. Interestingly, women who enjoy a few glasses of red wine with their food have higher sex drives and stronger orgasms, say Italian researchers. Eating boosts endorphins, the feel good hormones, while the antioxidants in red wine widen blood vessels, increasing blood flow to key sexual areas.[62]

Aphrodisiacs

Do you like seafood? Here's something you can enjoy—lobster. It's a rich source of zinc, important for the male libido as well as healthy sperm. Lobster is also a great source of protein, which boosts levels of dopamine and norepinephrine—two brain chemicals that heighten sensitivity during sex. The same food chemistry applies to oysters, which is why these shelled creatures are frequently referred to as an aphrodisiac.

Speaking of aphrodisiacs, among the many stories associated with all sorts of libido-raising foods, from ground rhino horn to cucumber, there are also aphrodisiac experiences associated with the other senses! These include things like the smell of freshly mown grass, the scent of the seaside and the smell of cucumber, of course. We mustn't forget our sight. Who hasn't had a naughty thought when seeing a banana! We also all have our favorite personalities who turn us on with their sexy voice.

Chocolate

Chocolate makes some women swoon at the very thought of it. Call it an aphrodisiac or not, it is rich in flavonoids—antioxidants—which are good for the heart and circulation. Flavonoids are also found in:

- Apples,
- Apricots,
- Blueberries,
- Pears,
- Raspberries,
- Strawberries,
- Black beans,
- Cabbage,
- Onions,
- Parsley,
- Pinto beans, and
- Tomatoes.

Chocolate is one of the most common cravings, particularly among women. This is because chocolate contains the same chemical—phenylethylamine—your brain creates when we're feeling romantic love. This is why many of us turn to chocolate when we are in need of love or feeling disappointed in a relationship.

What's more, the high fat content also soothes feelings of emptiness, insecurity or loneliness, while the texture can be creamy if you need comfort or crunchy if you're angry.

Chocolate also contains a serotonin-like substance called diphenylamine, which appears to promote feelings of calm. If our serotonin and energy levels are drained by stress-filled days, too-tight schedules, unhealthy eating, and lack of exercise, we often turn to chocolate to feel better. The stimulants in chocolate also act as an instant pick-me-up. Finally, pyrazine, a chemical found in chocolate odor, triggers the pleasure center in the brain.

So how do you beat your chocolate cravings? Ginger ale and soy milk have a high tyramine content, which can relieve chocolate cravings. The sweeteners in diet drinks stimulate brain production of phenylethylamine, the same "love-drug" found in chocolate, while the smell of coffee can alleviate chocolate cravings because it contains the same chemical (pyrazine) as chocolate.

Non-fat chocolate (frozen yogurt or fat-free brownies) may help, but be warned: fat-free doesn't necessarily mean low-calorie. Finally, aerobic exercise will boost serotonin levels, improve your mood and suppress appetite.[63]

Tomatoes

Tomatoes are rich in lycopene, the cancer-fighting phytonutrient, which is widely claimed to help prevent many cancers, including prostate, bladder and cervix. Plus, a review in the journal, *Food Research International,* suggests saffron, the yellow spice commonly used in Spanish, Indian and Italian cuisine, and ginseng are both natural aphrodisiacs.[64]

Supplements

Testosterone

"Testosterone is the main hormone that controls sexual desire, but the level slowly declines with age," says Dr. John Tomlinson, a general medical practitioner specializing in male sexual health and trustee of the Sexual Advice Association. "A man in his 70s has only two-thirds of the testosterone he had in his 20s.[65]

"Some men will find they just don't 'feel right;' they feel tired, crabby, their sex drive has diminished and if they take a Viagra-like tablet (Viagra itself, Cialis or Levitra), it doesn't always work properly. Although it tackles the mechanics of erectile dysfunction by improving blood flow, it doesn't boost testosterone and, therefore, desire."[66]

"It's worth noting two-thirds of men with erectile dysfunction have early onset coronary heart disease, in which no other symptoms, such as chest pain, are present," said Dr. Graham Jackson, consultant cardiologist to several London hospitals and with a practice on Harley Street, London, England.[67]

"Diabetes, thyroid disease and pituitary disease can also cause problems in the bedroom," Dr, Jackson continued, "so if you have a problem with erectile dysfunction, see your GP [medical practitioner] to have a testosterone test and rule these out."[68]

Testosterone has a strong influence on the libido of both men and women. Yes, although it is described as a male hormone, women, albeit in much smaller measure, also have testosterone. A simple blood test is all that is required. As your testosterone levels can vary greatly during the course of a day, be sure to have your test taken first thing in the morning. I should add, it is fairly uncommon for people to have lower than normal levels, but if this is the case, appropriate steps or treatment can be prescribed.

Testosterone deficiency is usually treated with testosterone replacement, available in a number of formulations including transdermal gel, patches, long and short-acting injections, oral treatment, and subcutaneous implants. Your medical practitioner will check you out for other possible causes and may even suggest certain lifestyle changes to affect a cure. Regular exercise and a healthy diet are may be all that is needed.

Zinc

Zinc has many functions in the body and contributes toward a healthy immune system. It is also known to help in fertility and reproduction, as pointed out by Dr. Christian Jessen.[69]

Iron

A low libido may be caused by an iron deficiency. Iron is crucial for transporting oxygen around the body, so anemia triggers excess tiredness, which can lead to lack of sex drive—low libido.[70] The condition can be detected through a blood test and treated with iron supplements. You can also combat anemia by ensuring your diet is complete with iron—rich foods including: spinach, sweet potatoes, beef, tofu, shrimp, tuna, beans, and a wide variety of other foods.

L-Arginine

L-Arginine is an amino acid, which is naturally combined with oxygen in the body to make nitric oxide. Amino acids are important for human metabolism and are the building blocks that link together to form proteins. One of L-Arginine's most important functions is its use in the synthesis of nitric oxide within the body. Nitric oxide acts as a signaling molecule and is involved in a variety of biological processes, most notably circulation to the extremities—especially the penis.

Lycopene

Lycopene is a natural ingredient found in many fruit and vegetables. Lycopene gives the strong red color to tomatoes. Studies suggest diets rich in tomatoes may account for lowering the risk of cancers of the lung, stomach and prostate. It may also help protect against cancer of the cervix, breast, mouth, pancreas, esophagus, colon, and rectum[71]. Although we're talking about supplements here, it is worth noting studies have suggested cooked tomatoes are more readily ingested by the small intestine than supplements in pill form.[72]

Read more about the benefits of lycopene here:

http://www.cancer.org/treatment/treatmentsandsideeffects/complementarya ndalternativemedicine/dietandnutrition/lycopene

Saw Palmetto

Saw palmetto is a plant, best known for decreasing prostate size in men suffering from BPH (benign prostatic hypertrophy). Nobody knows why the prostate gland increases in size as men get older, but it is a fact it does. Saw palmetto doesn't actually shrink the overall size of the prostate, but it does seem to shrink the inner lining that puts pressure on the urethra passing urine through the prostate. Saw palmetto supplements are made up of an extract of the plant and often blended with vitamins. It is also used by men who believe it has properties as an aphrodisiac.

Read more about saw palmetto here:

http://www.webmd.com/vitamins-supplements/ingredientmono-971-SAW %20PALMETTO.aspx? activeIngredientId=971&active IngredientName=SAW%20PALMETTO

Fenugreek

Fenugreek is a herb grown throughout Asia and is used most often to add flavor to curry dishes and other Indian recipes. Researchers from the Centre for Integrative Clinical and Molecular Medicine, in Brisbane, Australia, found men taking fenugreek can boost their sex drive by at least 25 percent.[73]

Sixty healthy men, between the ages of 25 and 52, took an extract of the herb twice a day for six weeks. Their libido levels were monitored using a scoring system to assess any changes after three and six weeks. Within six weeks, their scores had increased by an average of 28 percent. Concurrently, another group of men acting as a control group for comparison was fed a placebo. They saw their scores fall.[74]

Fenugreek seeds contain compounds called saponins, which are thought to stimulate production of male sex hormones including testosterone. One of the researchers noted, "This study has demonstrated that there was significant improvement in sexual function and performance following treatment."[75]

Ginseng

Ginseng has been used in the Far East for thousands of years to improve overall health. It is a fleshy root herb containing saponins that, like fenugreek, increases blood flow. There have been many studies carried out that indicate this herb can help impotence, but these studies are usually carried out experimentally on mice.

More recently, a study was carried out on 100 men by researchers at Yonsei University College of Medicine in South Korea. They found those with mild to moderate erectile dysfunction saw a small but significant improvement after taking Korean ginseng berry, four times a day for eight weeks[76].

Experts told the *International Journal of Impotence Research*, "Korean ginseng berry improved all domains of sexual function. It can be used as an alternative medicine to improve sexual life in men."[77]

Yohimbine

A therapy using bark from the yohimbe tree is hotly debated by bodybuilders and gym enthusiasts. Yohimbine is believed to increase blood flow to the genital area and prevent it from leaving too quickly.

You can read more about yohimbine at:

http://www.drugs.com/cdi/yohimbine.html#wIrZ2j1QqDMug7St.99

WARNING!!

The foregoing is a short list of supplements. They are mentioned here, because they are of general and sexual interest. There are many other herbal treatments commonly used with varying results. It is important you know these substances, in addition to the great many other alternative treatments available, can have a deleterious effect on your health and well being. In worst case scenarios, they can even cause death, if you do not seek personal medical advice before self-administering.

Some medical conditions may interact with supplements even herbal, 'organic,' or compound chemicals. Tell your doctor or pharmacist if you have any medical conditions before buying or taking supplementary treatments. Especially (but not limited to) if any of the following apply to you:

- If you are taking any prescription or non-prescription medicine, herbal preparation or dietary supplement.

- If you have allergies to medicines, foods or other substances.

- If you have a history of heart problems, kidney problems, high blood pressure, angina (chest pain), stomach or intestinal ulcers, or liver disease.

Oral Contraceptives

Although not a supplement, it's important to note the effect oral contraceptives can also have on your libido. "Ironically, many contraceptive pills can be passion killers," says women's health expert and nutritionist Dr. Marilyn Glenville. She goes on to say, "The hormones in the Pill trick your body into thinking you're already pregnant and don't need to reproduce. Also, by preventing ovulation, the Pill lowers levels of sexual desire and arousal."[78]

You can learn more about Dr. Glenville at

http://www.marilynglenville.com/about-dr-glenville/.

9

The Female Orgasm

An orgasm a day keeps the doctor away.

~ Mae West

When I asked my doctor for an exact description of the 'Big-O' he said,

> *The physiology of the orgasm is simply an explosion of nerve endings at the spinal cord level, without any brain activity, caused by stimulating the clitoris and glans to orgasm, at the very oldest part of the neurological system.*

Perhaps that's the biology behind the orgasm, but I think you'll agree that there's rather more to it than that. My research into the orgasm, has found more interesting answers!

I'm not disputing my medical practitioner's description. I'm certain he's given us a clue as to why women love to have their backs gently massaged, especially fingers running down the spine. Descriptions and opinions vary from woman-to-woman. To see and hear six women openly discussing what it feels like to have an orgasm, and the different types of orgasm each has experienced, take a few minutes to watch this short video found on Jason Julius' blog:

http://www.jasonjulius.com/the-female-orgasm-from-a-womans—perspective-what-it-feels-like/

As interesting as the comments from these six women are, it still leaves us with the question "How do I get to have orgasms like that?" and "What does my boyfriend have to do to get me to that point?"

Before I describe the different types of orgasm and how to achieve them, we should recognize any orgasm is the result of time taken in foreplay. However, even that is not as straightforward as the word "foreplay" implies. Foreplay includes a variety of components, including: emotional involvement, passion, the situational setting, opportunity, and most importantly communication.

Here's what Batwoman has to say on the subject,

> *Lovemaking technique, patience, (and) knowing about a lady's body and how to excite her (is needed to) bring her to orgasm in different ways. An empathy quotient and self-control play into this too. I like an adventuresome lover, with a sense of humor—a man who is willing to try new things to please me and to encourage me to try new things to please him. I want long, sexy lovemaking sessions where we both use our hands and mouths all over each other. I want him to love to look at my body, stroke me and sometimes bring me to orgasm with his fingers. When we get to intercourse, I want it to last awhile, and I don't want it to be in the same position every time. I want to feel passion and urgency sometimes—patience and humor at other times.*

What Batwoman describes is a major challenge for many men. However you can see how these desires work both ways for both men and women.

To better understand what's going on in the minds of men, *Cosmopolitan's* 'sexpert,' Rachel Morris, looked back at emails from male readers and told her female readers how to handle their most common sex worries. She brings to light some very good points women need to keep in mind, if they want to spice up their love life. These include:

- **Taking Charge**—It's not always the man's job to take the lead in your physical relationship. Don't be afraid of being in charge sometimes and initiating sex.

- **The Orgasm Enigma**—For men, the female orgasm can be harder to figure out than a Rubick's Cube. With so many different ways a woman can orgasm, and the fact that sometimes something works better than at other times, it's no wonder men get confused. Be sure to let your man know what you like and give gentle guidance to help him get you there.

- **Don't Let Societal Stigmas Hamper Your Sex Life**— Although Morris specifically talks about sharing your submission fantasies with your partner, and allowing them to sometimes let their inner caveman out, this also holds true for other fantasies and fetishes you may have, but are afraid "nice girls don't do that." Talk to your partner. If it's consensual and no one is harmed, you never know what heights you can achieve until you try. Read more about this topic in Chapter 21: Fetish and Fantasy.

- **Performance Anxiety**—The penis can be a great anxiety barometer in men. If they're worried about performing, or have other anxiety issues, it may result in erectile dysfunction, premature ejaculation, or even not being able to orgasm at all. If this happens, be understanding and don't show your frustration, your frustration will only make him more anxious and compound the problem in the future.

- **It's a Guy Thing**—One common complaint men have is their partner's libido isn't as active as theirs. They also are more inclined to want "foreplay-free quickies," where women often prefer sex that's more involved. These different gender preferences aren't something you can help; however, if your man has gone out of his way to satisfy you in bed, remember to reciprocate in kind sometimes, to let him know how much you appreciate him.[79]

Morris has summed up some important points nicely on how a woman can help her man give her the best orgasms. Later, I flesh this topic out more fully, so that both men and women can understand the cause and effect of the orgasm, and employ fully described techniques, to reach the greatest heights of sexual fulfillment, with the most powerful orgasmic experiences. Guys, this isn't just for women.

Learn to Love Your Body!

One strong aspect of sex, for the male particularly, is the visual component. A man can be turned on simply by seeing the female form. Females know this. This is why they pay so much attention to the way they look. For the same reason, women often have doubts about their physical shape and, because of this, some prefer to make love in the dark, so their partner doesn't have to look at them.

If you are a woman and this is something you've been thinking, I want to dispel the myth right now. 'Looks' don't factor into the equation much, if at all, when the chemistry of lust and the emotional bond of love kick in.

Here's something you can do the next time you're alone and naked in the bedroom. Place a mirror on the floor and squat over it, with your knees apart. Look down and you will see the reflection in the mirror of your vulva—that's all the 'bits' between your legs. This is the picture your lover will find so irresistible. He can't wait to get down to it!

Great Sex Has Nothing to do with Perfect Bodies

Dr. Barbara Bartlik, renowned integrative psychiatrist and sex therapist, cautions people to not worry so much about our flaws. By constantly focusing on your fat bottom or love handle, or whatever other physical flaw you feel you have, it's going to damage your sex drive. Instead, Dr. Bartlik recommends thinking about your body from your partner's perspective and remember that these perceived flaws have never prevented your partner from loving every moment they get to spend with you having sex.[80]

Men may be picky about women's bodies on TV; however, when it comes to real life, great sex has nothing to do with perfect bodies. At the first sign you're becoming self-consciousness during sex, turn off your brain and concentrate on how sensual your body feels and how into it your partner is. The sound of his breathing, the way your bodies fit together—keep your focus on the physical to put you in a more passionate mental state. You'll forget about everything else.

I want that to sink in. It's going to be very relevant when we get to the 'hot' stuff, so read that last paragraph again.

The Benefits of Orgasms

As an interesting side note—orgasms can help you stay slim. Orgasms trigger the production of phenethylamine, a chemical messenger in the brain that regulates appetite. In addition, 50% of female migraine sufferers find their symptoms were reduced after orgasm.[81] It's thought endorphins released during sex closely resemble morphine and act in a similar way.

The Biggest Sex Organ

For women the best aphrodisiacs are words. The G-spot is in the ears. He who looks for it below there is wasting his time.

~ Isabel Allende

Neuroscientist Barry Komisaruk, of Rutgers University, discovered from his research into the neuroscience of the female orgasm in 2011, the biggest sexual organ could well be the brain. In the name of science, he persuaded several broad-minded women to agree to be strapped into a MRI scanner to have their brain patterns monitored while they climaxed. The study revealed an explosion of activity across 30 areas of the brain. Surprisingly, this was also the case in individuals who can achieve orgasm by thought alone![82]

Kayt Sukel, science writer and sex expert, believes women are able to experience a feeling of sexual arousal every bit as easily and intensely as a man can. "In short," she says, "the female orgasm is much more complicated and less predictable than it was believed."[83]

In her book, Sukel notes that one of the areas of the brain stimulated by orgasm is the prefrontal cortex, which is the part of the brain that controls complex functions including—imagination, controlling urges and making decisions.[84] Sukel understands that both sexes are capable of achieving orgasm by thought alone (although I also believe you have to be very physically fit to do this, which is probably why you may only hear of men and women under the age of 30 with this ability.)

In contrast, the team of researchers from the University of Groningen, in the Netherlands, led by Janniko Georgiadis found far from lighting up like a Christmas tree, the same brain region in women 'switched off' when they were reaching orgasm with a partner.

It is possible there is a difference between someone trying to mentalize sexual stimulation, as opposed to receiving it from a partner. I don't think orgasm turns off consciousness, but it changes it. When you ask people how they perceive their orgasm, they describe a feeling of a loss of control. I'm not sure if this altered state is necessary to achieve more pleasure or is just some side-effect," says Janniko Georgiadis.[85]

The implication is women's brains behave differently when experiencing pleasure, according to whether they are alone or with a partner. It also suggests a woman's solo orgasm may be different to the one she experiences with another person.

Another thing to add to the complexities—a woman's sex drive peaks in the evening because her levels of sex hormone, progesterone, are highest at this time. Unfortunately, a man's sex drive is greatest in the morning, as his levels of testosterone build up overnight.

Female Physiology

There are a variety of methods that can cause female orgasm, as listed below. To better understand why this stimulation works, we need to know the location of the various parts that can trigger an orgasm. Although the basic result is "an explosion of nerve endings at spinal cord level without any brain activity," as the doctor told us at the beginning of this chapter, the physical stimulation can be coupled with brain activity to produce differing levels of 'explosion.'

The variety of stimulation that can cause orgasm, includes:

- Unintentional stimulation, through sporting exercise,

- Masturbation, solo

- Masturbation, by your partner—including oral

- Clitoral, through clitoral contact during penetrative sex

- Vaginal, through contact with 'G-spot' area

- Vaginal, through contact with 'A-spot' area

- Anal, by stimulation of the 'A-spot' through the wall of the rectum

Before you leap to your keyboard and start listing other areas not on this list, and before I begin to describe techniques using hands, fingers, lips, tongue, hair, etc, we need to know where the most densely-populated and most sensitive nerve areas are located.

Inside the Female Reproductive System

When it comes to sexual stimulation, there are plenty of other places that can come into play, like the mouth, ears, neck, breasts, nipples, underarms, forearms, tummy, thighs, knees, and feet. Let's identify the most important parts first. We'll be talking about those other places later. Right now, let's take a look inside the female reproductive system. (See Figure 5: Cross-Section Female Reproductive System, in Chapter 3.)

The G-Spot

About 2 inches (50mm) inside the vagina, and situated on its front wall, is the G-Spot. This area, which to the touch feels like the surface of a sponge is commonly about the size of a small coin. It is what is left of what would have been the prostate gland in the male. There has been much debate about this gland, ranging from denial of its existence to it being the source of the strongest orgasmic experiences.

In 2001, the Federative Committee on Anatomical Terminology accepted 'female prostate' as an accurate term for the Skene's gland, also known as the G-Spot. First discovered by Regnier de Graaf, who was the first to hypothesize about this equivalent to a man's prostate. 'G-Spot' was coined in 1981 and named after the German gynecologist, Ernst Grafenberg, who re-discovered this marvelous spot.

So much has been written about the G-spot and whether it really exists or is just a figment of imagination of fertile minds. When Batwoman was asked for an opinion, here's what she said, "I have a G—spot. It took years and the right guy to find it, but it is there, and it is a whole lot of fun."

From Fig.5 on Page 20, you can also see the female urethra is quite short, unlike a man's urethra, which is as long as his penis plus the distance within his body before it connects to his bladder. In a woman, the urethra is about 1.5 inches (35mm) long. This is one reason why females are more prone to cystitis than males; proximity to the outside of the body lends itself to increased chance of infection.

Another small area, only about 1 inch (25mm) in size, is the distance between the lower end of the vulva and the anus. As our family doctor once said, "You have to remember that the playground is only an inch away from the sewer!" Obviously, personal hygiene is important; however, the vagina is self-cleaning. Don't douche (unless directed to do so by a healthcare practitioner); it's not necessary. Just keep the vulva washed and clean.

Ladies First

Nine Plus One: A Chinese Way of Thrusting

The man does nine shallow thrusts and one deep. He then does eight shallow thrusts and two deep. Next is seven shallow thrusts and three deep, etc. until one shallow thrust and nine deep. Fellas, see if you can last that long. For men, counting makes them last longer, while for women the variation of pattern heightens sensitivity.

~ Sex Again: Recharging Your Libido by Jill Blakeway

Guys, if you're a man who believes and practices the theory that his woman should be allowed to climax before he does, here's a way of making this courtesy even better for your partner.

Following whatever is your usual or favored warm up and foreplay, take it to the next level with penetrative sex. Bring her close to climax, then slow down the rhythm, so she doesn't cum. Communication is key with this. You both need to know what stage you're at. Slowly raise the rhythm again until she approaches her climax once more.

It is very hard for her to resist letting go at this stage, but believe me she will feel the strength of her desire to orgasm growing with each stage of holding off. It's very much like when a man edges: getting closer to ejaculation but stopping short before it happens.

When she decides enough is enough, and tells you she is going to cum, let her do it. You, the man, continue thrusting until her orgasm begins to subside. At this point, only a few seconds after her orgasm, withdraw your penis just enough, so you are rubbing her G-spot (about 2 inches inside the front wall of her vagina) with your penis head and ejaculate over this spot.

It takes a strong will to let it go, denying the natural instinct to thrust in as deep as you can at this point, but that's what you need to do. If you are blessed with a larger than average penis, you may find it necessary to hold your penis in one hand to make sure you hit the spot. Because this part of the vagina is rich in sensitive nerve endings, she will feel it when you cum. The warm fluid being rubbed into her G-spot by your penis will often bring her to a second climax almost immediately.

Don't worry if it doesn't the first time you try. You will both have enjoyed a sensual and satisfying coupling.

Female Ejaculation

With practice, the tension of building up to this point will give her stronger and stronger orgasms. At a further stage in your experimenting with this, she might even get the feeling she wants to pee as she climaxes. This is a magic moment, and one that requires courage the first time. Let me explain.

She remembers emptying her bladder before this session. It doesn't feel right to let go and urinate on you anyway, so she Kegels and holds off peeing. If she holds off what she thinks might be pee, she will be missing a golden opportunity to hit a real high spot in climaxing. The timing of this need-to-pee feeling, coinciding with the direct stimulation of her G—spot by your penis, lubricated with semen, means a vaginal orgasm is about to happen. Her G-spot produces a fluid—not unlike your pre-cum, and certainly not like urine, and needs her urethra open to let it out.

Here's what she needs to do. Instead of clamping off to prevent what she feels is peeing, she has to do the absolute reverse. She opens up her urethra and pushes down just like she does when wanting to expel as much urine and as fast as possible. Only this time it is not urine. As I said, the first time takes courage, but she will know if it is a vaginal orgasm because firstly it will be an incredibly strong climax—quite possibly making her physically shake—and, secondly, you will both notice an increased wetness.

When you have successfully achieved this type of heightened orgasm, it is not uncommon for the woman to want to continue being stimulated to further orgasms straight away. By this time, you would probably have to stimulate her using your fingers and her vulva would be visible to you. As she pushes down you might notice her whole vulva swelling in time with her rhythmic contractions and the G-spot fluid flowing out. The amount of fluid varies from woman to woman. With some, it is just extra wetness, with others it can be enough to enable her to squirt. Squirting is an amazing feeling for the woman and an equally amazing sight for the man.

Be experimental, be open-minded, be patient, but do try it out. For ladies who cum first, this can also become ladies who cum and cum and cum!

—— 10 ——

Vaginal Orgasm

The only thing wrong with being an atheist is that there's nobody to talk to during an orgasm.

~ Author Unknown

If you are a woman reading this book, I'd like to apologize for the fact there's no way I can write about techniques without being absolutely clinical. I know this isn't the sort of thing that springs to mind when you're enjoying yourself; however, knowledge is power. In the case of trying to 'get there,' an understanding of what is happening will help you help yourself, as well as help your partner, to arrive at the gate of the amazing sex a vaginal orgasm will bring.

Going for a G-Spot Orgasm

If you are a man reading this book, I make no apologies for the fact going for the gold of a G-spot vaginal orgasm is going to be a selfless act of the highest order. In other words, forget about your own needs and concentrate entirely on hers. You will, I promise, not only enjoy the exercise, you will also feel the erotic impact on your own body, which hearing and seeing a woman cum in this way can have.

It doesn't stop there. As you both progress toward her achieving an ejaculatory or squirting orgasm, you will enjoy the incredible sight of a woman in the throes of uncontrollable orgasmic contractions, which make her whole body shake with pleasure.

Before we go any further, do not expect immediate ultimate results. The most rewarding experiences result from discovering what works best for you and your woman. We're all different, and what triggers orgasms for one girl may not work for another. Pay careful attention to her reactions, make a mental note of what seems to spur her on, and never repeat mistakes! You can follow a rule book and get nowhere, and you can also be rewarded in just a few enlightened attempts. Just be patient, dedicated and loving.

In the lead-up to this, let her know this is going to be 'her time' and not to worry about you. You will get your reward later. Reassure her. She might think you are doing all the stimulating, but you will definitely be aroused. By the time she cums, your own level of excitement will be rising, and you will probably be able to ejaculate within seconds, if that is what you'd like to do.

A friend of mine, Roly, told me about the time his wife had a vaginal orgasm, in such a dramatic way, the sight and sound of this set him off so quickly, he decided to let his ejaculate fly at her breasts. The first spurt of his hot ejaculate hit one of her fully pert and erect nipples, and the unexpected surprise gave her a spontaneous orgasm. Two hot orgasms for her, within seconds of each other, and from two totally different erotic spots!

Remember to prepare. Well manicured hands and finger nails are very important. Create the ideal situation—a relaxing time with no chance of interruptions and wipes, lubricant and a spare pillow handy. Sooner or later, you are going to need a towel as well; more about that in a minute.

It would be good to talk about what you propose to treat her to several hours before or even the day before. Anticipation builds desire and excitement. Best of all, clear her mind of other things that would otherwise spoil the moment. Don't say you're going to give her a G-spot orgasm, even though this is what you will be aiming for, because she will feel like she has let you down if it doesn't happen. Worse still, she might pretend to have an orgasm, and both of you will never learn the true sublime satisfaction an actual G-spot orgasm can bring.

Much has been written about how much time you should spend on foreplay. Remember, foreplay can turn into a satisfying conclusion itself. The time required to move from foreplay to the all-consuming act of full, penetrative sex can vary from a couple of minutes to 20 minutes or more, depending on the circumstances and how ready through anticipation and desire she is to move her whole being into gear.

Locating the G-Spot

For this section, penile penetration is not going to play any part in her reaching orgasm, at least not right now. For this reason, you could call the technique I'm about to describe as simply extended foreplay.

You have already read and seen, in a diagrammatic cross-section of the female reproductive organs, where the vagina is situated relative to the other organs. For most of its length, about four inches (100mm) in its rested state, it has fewer sensory nerve endings than the skin on your arms. However, within the first two inches (50mm), it has an abundance of nerve endings, making it very sensitive. The final half-inch (10mm), at the deepest point, also has a significant number of nerve endings; we will talk about this 'A' spot later.

What is the G-Spot?

As we noted earlier, the G-spot is a tiny piece of tissue, rich in nerve endings, and is located about 1.5 to two inches (40 to 50mm) inside and on the front wall of the vagina. The Skene's Gland also covers this area and is there to provide lubrication within the vaginal walls. The G-spot varies in size from woman-to-woman and from age-to-age. It also seems to have an ability to increase in size for women who stimulate it on a regular basis.

There are more glands within the vagina. The Bartholin's glands are on both sides of the vagina, nearer the entrance. They exude lubricant at the entrance to the vagina and within the labia. When the female is excited, both these glands excrete lubricant to make entry for the penis easier. This is what is commonly referred to as 'being wet.'

Some women produce more natural lubricant than others. All women become 'dry' as they get older. The age at which this happens varies from woman-to-woman. This makes the application of external lubricants not only desirable but sensible, even for women who do not yet feel the need.

It is thought the Skene's gland also excretes fluid into the urethra. If liquid appears from the female urethra and is clear and virtually tasteless, this is not urine but instead female ejaculate.

Don't be Anxious

A short note of caution and reassurance is good at this point. There are many women who claim it took several months to find their G-spot, and there are others who are absolutely convinced they do not have one at all. To these women, I want to say you should never feel inadequate.

You are as normal as the next woman, even as normal as those who are able to orgasm this way and 'squirt' their ejaculate like a man squirts his. Paula Hall, a sex counselor, for UK Marriage and Relationship Counselling, said, "This kind of information is always interesting. If you have difficulties with your sex life, then a greater biological understanding might be helpful, but for some people it will create more anxiety."

Listen to what Batwoman has to say on the subject.

For me, the effects of G-spot stimulation are subtle at first. If I had someone saying, 'Is this it? How about here? Now do I have it?' and generally distracting me from relaxing and enjoying the sensations, well, I'm not sure we would ever have found my G. It took a while before I realized when he did certain things a certain way for long enough, then the sensations changed in what eventually added up to a dramatic way. This is one of those things that takes patience and time. It cannot be rushed or made into a stressful 'we must find it' sort of thing.'

Fingers do, indeed, work extremely well for G-spot stimulation. Once I learned what it felt like, I realized I could also guide my partner into positions that hit my G-spot better during (penile) sex, too.

G-spots may be hard to find, which is probably why many people don't think they are real. In my case, I wasn't sure if I had one or not until my partner and I made a really focused search for mine. The G-spot is not (for me, at least) a button you can push. Rather, it is an area that when stroked gives me a deeper, different form of arousal.

It does not have well-defined edges, but he can tell when he's there from my responses. Also, I believe, the texture is different and grows more different as I get more excited. Usually it takes some clitoral stimulation, in addition to my G-spot attention, to make me cum, but orgasms when he's been stroking my G-spot are almost always deeper and more powerful than I get from other activities, like oral or finger play without attention to my G-spot.'

Feeling a Need to Pee

When the feeling like you need to pee is really ejaculate, it's from a build up of fluid from the Skene's gland. It places pressure on the sphincter (the muscle you use to hold back urination) and produces this feeling of wanting to relieve pressure. However, if your woman has arrived at the point of orgasm and won't let it go, the fluid is simply forced back up and into the bladder, where it will stay until she next visits the toilet. If she often has to go pee as soon as your sexual activity has finished, it's probably the effect as I have described. What she is missing is the feeling of immense rush to orgasm produced by the fluid being forced, just like a man, out of her urethra by her orgasmic contractions.

As Batwoman notes,

> I know the 'need to pee' feeling. It comes from the fact some of the nerves that are involved are right next to the bladder. However, the feeling does not necessarily indicate she is going to pee if you keep rubbing her G-spot or if she cums. For me, the feeling (if I get it) goes away as I get closer to orgasm.

My advice is to talk to your girl and suggest she pee before you start anything. If she comes to bed with the confidence her bladder is completely empty, then maybe you can get her past the 'need to pee' feeling, so you can both enjoy some really big G-spot orgasms.

The Secret to Female Ejaculation

What happens most of the time, and for most but not all women, is you become suddenly aware of being a lot wetter around the vulva when you cum. When the female arrives at the need-to-pee feeling, instead of clamping shut, to avoid letting it go, you push down. Yes, imagine you've been dying to pee for so long when you finally get to a place where you can let go and your bladder is so full, you push down hard to expel the pee. It comes out in a jet-like stream. It's such a satisfying feeling, isn't it? Well, if you thought that was satisfying, wait until you 'squirt' your female ejaculate like that!

You may not actually squirt the first time or even after several times, but if and when you do, you will experience the kind of orgasm unlike anything else. You will want to do it again and again. The first few times you may just be aware of a greater degree of wetness than you have had before, but the intensity will be greater.

If you have any doubts about the fluid being female ejaculate, there are some distinct differences. First, pee smells. Second, it is most often colored—usually with a slight yellowish tinge. If your urine is ever a dark yellow, this is likely a sign you're dehydrated from not drinking enough fluids. Female ejaculate, on the other hand, has no odor, is a clear liquid but may be a tiny bit thicker in consistency to urine. This is similar in appearance and consistency to a man's 'pre-cum,' which is produced by the Cowper's Gland. Lastly, when female ejaculate is coming or 'squirting' you have absolutely no control over stopping it (not that you would want to because of the heightened pleasure it brings!)

NOTE: If you are having problems leaking urine, either at the point of penile penetration, approaching or during orgasm, this could be an indication of something else going on that needs attention. I'll be covering this and other similar topics, for both sexes, in Chapter 23: Problem Solving.

At the point of orgasm, as the ejaculate travels from the G-spot into and through the urethra and the woman pushes down, the man will feel the vagina trying to push his fingers out. When this happens during penetrative sex, he feels the vagina pushing his penis out. It's an extraordinary feeling for both partners.

With experience and practice, the female's whole-body orgasm stimulated this way will often produce contractions so strong they make her body shake. The emotional tie to the event can even bring her to tears, but in a good way—a very good way!

G-Spot Technique

With your partner lying on her back, you kneel comfortably beside her. I say 'comfortably,' because you could be in this position for up to 30 minutes. Place the spare pillow under her buttocks, so her whole pelvic region is raised. Do this together; she can lift herself while you slide the pillow underneath her. Spread her legs a little, so you have complete access to her vulva. She may raise her knees; this is okay, too. When she is close to orgasm, she may want to stretch her legs out straight, so make sure there's plenty of leg room for her.

Apply lubricant to the vulva, from the lower end to the clitoris at the top, and then some well into the entrance of her vagina. Slide the index finger of your dominant hand into her vagina, with the palm facing down. Point the finger down and then run it up along the side walls, first to one side then the other. This helps the muscles surrounding the vagina to relax. It's important not to go straight for the G-spot, just as you shouldn't go straight for the clitoris. These are sensitive places and need to be approached with loving tenderness.

Continue moving your finger around in this way for a couple of minutes, and then turn your hand around so the palm of your hand is now facing upwards. With the tip of your finger, you can now feel around the forward part of the vagina. Make small circular motions with the tip and, from a point as deep as you can get, start to withdraw your finger—but not completely.

What you are seeking is an area that feels different to the rest of the vagina wall. It's sometimes described as a 'spongy' area. It is not clearly defined, and it may be very small. It may also be slightly harder than the surrounding walls. When you have found the area with a different feel to it, make a 'come here' motion with your finger.

Don't rush it. Make the finger movement fairly slowly, no faster than one complete movement per second. Bring your finger firmly up against the front wall as though you are trying to hook her G-spot out of her vagina. Keep it slow, until her responses indicate speeding up would be good.

When she is completely relaxed, you can use two fingers. Remove the first and then re-enter with two. This will enable you to double up the 'come here' action, by alternating one finger to the next—a bit like walking your fingers but staying on the same spot. Although it's a little trickier than simply writing about it, it's very effective. Just watch her reaction!

If after approximately ten minutes you don't seem to be getting anywhere, get your head down over her pubis and lay your tongue across her clitoris. If she gives out a moan, or uses her hands to press your head harder against her, don't change what you are doing. It will lead to a satisfying conclusion. If, however, you know your woman so well you know it always takes her a long time to orgasm, try this:

- Press down on her pubic bone with the flat palm of your free hand, so it is being squeezed between your finger inside her vagina and your hand on the outside. This adds to the pressure your fingers can apply to her erogenous zone.

- Alternatively, if you find her G-spot is not so far inside her vagina, keep two fingers (middle and third) working, with the other two (index and little) pointing down, and bend your hand so the palm is pressing down on her clitoris.

- Holding this position, almost like a clamp, raise and lower your hand in a fairly fast motion, so both her G-spot and clitoris are being firmly shaken (but, please, not violent). When fully aroused, this action will give her multiple orgasms and a series of involuntary spasms that will shake her whole body—and the smile on her face will tell you she doesn't want to stop.

You will know when you've hit the spot, and she's becoming aroused, because the G-spot will harden and swell. It is not always apparent at first and often comes as a surprise (to both of you), as the swelling on the front wall expands and can push you out as she orgasms. Alternatively, she might just enjoy a less dramatic orgasm. If this is the case, your finger will feel a series of tiny contractions, sometimes described as butterflies.

Even when using plenty of lubricant, this exercise can make her vagina sore if continued for too long. No matter what age, never prolong the finger movement beyond 30 minutes.

Throughout this exercise, keep an eye on her reactions. If she is lying still tell her to breathe deeply. If her breathing becomes shallow, she could even fall asleep with the comforting and relaxing sensations she will be enjoying! Tell her how wonderful it is for you to be feeling inside her—and sharing this experience.

The A-Spot

The A-spot, what's the A-spot? If you're like many people, you've heard a lot about the G-spot but nothing about the A-spot. What is it? The term 'A-spot' is derived from the medical term— Anterior Fornix Erogenous zone, or AFE.

Research on this erogenous zone has been sporadic and made by only a handful of scientists. There have been several papers published on the subject, mostly by 'sex experts,' and opinions have been given by many others who claim to not only identify this spot but also how to stimulate it. Being a little skeptical, I note those who make such claims have not, so far, freely published their techniques for all to follow but provide the information only upon payment.

Following you'll find resources centering on the who, the why and the how of A-spot research, so, if you wish to go for an A-spot vaginal orgasm, you will have as much information as necessary to achieve it.

A-Spot Research

Dr. Chua Chee Ann has a Masters in Public Health, with a sub—specialization in Sexual Health. In his research with female subjects suffering from vaginal dryness, Dr. Ann found stimulating an area deep in the vagina on the anterior wall resulted in rapid lubrication and arousal. Dr. Ann promotes his A-spot stimulation techniques in books and at seminars. You can see a video where he was interviewed about his work at www.aspot-pioneer.com.

His technique involves applying pressure to the area, making a scooping motion and stimulating other parts of the vagina. Dr. Ann claims, if practiced for at least ten minutes a day, it will make vaginal lubrication and orgasms regularly attainable, even without foreplay. Indeed, he even goes on to say lubrication can be achieved within five to ten seconds and orgasm in as little as two minutes! You can read a transcript of his interview at http://www.aspot-pioneer.com/pdf/DrChuaInterviewScript.pdf

There is some disagreement between exponents regarding A-spot stimulation. Some say the zone we're interested in is located at the deepest point of the vagina, on its anterior wall, above the cervix, where the vagina starts to curve upwards. Others describe it as being on the posterior wall of the vagina, approximately opposite the G-spot. Dr. Ann disagrees with this, while yet another belief is this area may be a different erogenous zone altogether!

From these confusing opinions, I think you will agree while we wait for further studies, you and I should make our own discoveries and see just what we can achieve for ourselves and our partners.

Locating the A-Spot

Toward the deepest point of the vagina, on its anterior (or forward) side, is the cervix. It is through the center of the cervix where sperm must travel, in order to reach the uterus. It is surrounded by the *fornix*—Latin for 'arch', which is an appropriate description for the form it takes around the cervix.

In most women, the cervix is extremely sensitive. I know of women who have fainted when their cervix has been touched. However, because of the position of the fornix, there are two areas that interest us—the deepest part of the vagina immediately before the fornix and, because it is possible to pass beyond the cervix to the end of the vagina, an area variously described as the 'deep spot,' 'cul-de-sac' or 'rectouterine pouch.' This is possibly another erogenous zone altogether. Theories abound, but there is a belief that material, as found in the Skene's gland and the G-spot glands, might also be found in the area where the vaginal nerves connect. This would explain the spontaneous excretion of lubricating fluid when the A-spot area is stimulated.

A-Spot Technique

To keep it simple, I will refer to the anterior spot as the A-spot on the front wall and the posterior position as the back of the A-spot. Women who enjoy orgasms resulting from stimulation of this erogenous zone claim they are more 'intense' than orgasms produced by clitoral stimulation.

Taking up Dr. Ann's technique described as a scooping motion, imagine you have just finished a fruit salad topped with cream. There's a little a little cream left in the bottom of the bowl, so you dip your middle (longest) finger into the bottom of the bowl. With a scooping motion, your finger runs around the bottom of the bowl and picks up the remaining cream. Use this analogy for stimulating the A-spot.

Whether it's the anterior or posterior side at the end of her vagina, the scooping motion, with your longest finger, is likely to cover both. If one creates a bigger reaction than the other, I don't have to tell you where to concentrate!

It's interesting to note Dr. Ann mentions he discovered stimulating two areas of the vagina at the same time produced the quickest lubrication and fastest orgasm. If, without resorting to a toy, you can find a way of stimulating her A-spot at the same time as her G-spot, you're in for the most dramatic and intense orgasm a woman can have. The only way I can find to achieve such a move is with full penetrative penile sex—to be covered under the section on Best Positions.

For your first try, using the middle finger of your dominant hand, your partner should lie on her back with a pillow under her buttocks and her legs over her head. Insert your finger with palm down to target her posterior fornix zone or with palm facing up for her anterior spot. With this latter position, your index and third fingers will be pointing up and away from her vagina. Use these fingers to squeeze her labia together; this will send signals back up to her clitoris. A combination of clitoral and vaginal orgasm is going to make her go wild.

Your longest finger may not reach her A-spot. Your fingers may be short or her vagina too long. The length of vaginas vary as much as the length of mens penises. For this reason, I'll be offering variations in positions for all to try.

— 11 —

Men Faking It

*Men don't fake orgasm—no man wants to
pull a face like that on purpose.*

~ Allan Pease

Although body language expert and motivational speaker, Allan Pease, was kidding when he said the above quote, the reality is—men do sometimes fake orgasm. However, before we get into the male side of this topic, let's begin with the ladies.

Women Faking It

We've all seen the famous film clip of Sally, played by Meg Ryan, in the romantic comedy film *When Harry Met Sally.* She gets the attention of not only her good friend, Harry, played by Billy Crystal, but also the entire cafe, when she demonstrates how effectively she can fake an orgasm. "I'll have what she's having!" a fellow cafe patron quips.

It has become generally accepted fact women can and do fake orgasms, and they might do so for a number of reasons.

- Perhaps she's tired but doesn't want to upset her partner or disappoint him.

- She may fake it just to get the encounter over with as quickly as possible, so she can turn over and get some sleep.

- Maybe she feels insecure and fears her partner might stray if he thinks he can't get her to orgasm every time.

- Maybe she's simply not going to get there, for any number of reasons, and knows it's just easier to fake it, rather than hurt her partner's feelings.

As we get older and our relationship matures, with the knowledge achieving orgasm every time is wonderful but not absolutely essential—the wanting to hold each other close, and doing so, being just as important—thinking we might fake an orgasm doesn't even cross our mind. If orgasm happens, fine. If it doesn't, we are still able to express our love. If, at this stage, the woman still thinks she needs to fake it, she should talk it over with her partner or seek counseling.

However, in early and mid-life encounters, both sexes set out to please and satisfy their partners. A major part of the satisfaction is the ability to bring about a climax.

Stories of women trying to avoid sex—"I've got a headache" or "I'm too tired" or "I've got to be up early in the morning" abound. This has become so prevalent, men have come to accept the fact a woman doesn't always want sex. If she fails to convince him she's really not in the mood, she may fake an orgasm to get it over quickly and hope he won't be disappointed.

The Sexual Shift

The emphasis on who is demanding sex is shifting. Until recent generations, it has always been the man who has initiated sex. However, with women discovering greater freedom in all aspects of their lives, it's become more socially acceptable for them to feel comfortable asking for and initiating sex. No longer just the meek housewives, women are finally embracing their sexuality.

There is an ongoing power shift between men and women in the wider world that has led to role reversal in the bedroom. In some instances, it can create a masculinity crisis for men. This is compounded by the increasing numbers of women who have become the main breadwinner in their households. These psychological battles often have physiological outcomes. The man may not feel like having sex when he feels his masculinity is threatened.

For this reason, the pressure is on. Men are finding themselves in situations where they are expected to perform, even if they are not feeling up to it.

It's expected men will understand if a woman declines an opportunity to have sex. It has always been understood when a woman expresses her emotional wishes, the man should respect these. Despite this, as recently as the 1950's, society used the term "wifely duty." The wife had little choice. It was actually assumed women didn't enjoy sex, but rather they had to submit to it for the benefit of the marital relationship.

Emotional avoidance also comes into play. Even as a boy, I, like many other men, was taught to hide my emotions. "Strong men don't cry," I was told as a kid. The 'stiff upper lip' was a very British guidance for all boys and young men, if they ever dared to show emotion. This attitude isn't only Brits; it is ingrained in the minds of many men universally. If a man would prefer to decline sex, he must 'put on a brave face' and get on with it.

Men are always expected to want sex, so they're not used to explaining if they don't want to do something—and worry their partner will think less of them.

How Does He Fake It?

Just how do men fake it? Given the obvious result when a man climaxes, how does he fake an orgasm without ejaculating?

When using a condom, it is easy to hide the fact he hasn't orgasmed. The man is expected to go to the bathroom to dispose of it following a climax. However, even with unprotected sex, as we will learn from 'A Woman's Perspective', the woman doesn't usually feel the actual ejaculate, just the tensing of the man's frame as he climaxes and perhaps the pulsing that comes with ejaculation. A few well-timed Kegels can mimic this pulsing.

As far as the ejaculate itself, the woman's own juices make her wet, so it can become indistinguishable, and she may not realize there is anything amiss. However, semen does have a very distinctive smell. A woman with a sensitive nose may notice the lack of smell, even if you pretend to ejaculate inside of her. This may be particularly true, if she's cleaning up after sex. Interestingly, there has yet to be a survey conducted about women who have discovered their men faking it.

Faked Orgasms: The Reality

The expectation men are always in the mood for sex, and are also capable of providing endless explosive sexual experiences, is another reason why men may increasingly want to fake an orgasm. A men's website, Askmen.com, conducted a survey of 2,000 men in 2012, They found 34 percent admitted faking it. This is up from 17 percent in 2010.[86]

In their 2013 survey, having asked the similar question, *Have you ever faked an orgasm during intercourse?*, the number remained at 34 percent. They added a response choice: *Yes, on more than one occasion*, the number was 20 percent. For the answer choice, *Yes, but only once*, 14 percent responded positively.[87]

A survey of more than 200 college students, published in *The Journal of Sex Research,* found that in addition to approximately half of women admitting they had faked an orgasm, 25 percent of the male college students said they had faked it. The study found that the most common motivation for faking it was "wanting sex to end without the awkwardness of hurting their partner's feelings."[88]

Harvard Professor Dr Abraham Morgentaler, author of *Why Men Fake It: The Totally Unexpected Truth About Man and Sex*, was interviewed on the Moll Flanders Show. He said, "Men fake it when they think orgasm isn't going to happen—the same as women do." He went on to say, "Men want to be gallant or noble but don't always know what it is that their woman wants. They want to feel valued."[89]

Moll Flanders asked if Dr Abraham Morgentaler could provide five points to help women understand the situation. Below is an extract of the dialogue in that interview:

- Men want to be manly. So sometimes what that means is let the guy make the decision, even if you think you know what's right. There are ways women can get what they want and still let the guy feel he's the decider (if you will) and everybody wins.

- Understand that the man wants to be a provider in bed. So it's not whatever you've read in girl's magazines and whatever you've heard from girlfriends is not true. If he wants to do something that is really nice for you, let him.

- Men are people too. By that what I mean is that they've got feelings even though they've been trained their whole life to try and not show them. So I think that it is really easy, when someone doesn't give you much emotion back, to try and get a rise out of somebody. The guys feel cutting comments just like your best girlfriends do.

- A little compliment for a guy goes an awful long way. For a woman to tell the man something—it can be small, like 'you look really good in that shirt', or after sex, for example, even better, like,'mmm, that was great.' (At this point Moll Anderson interjects with, "Or, you rock my world! Does that work?" 'Perfect", replies Dr Morgentaler). You can do that once a week and the guy will be on cloud nine.

- I think that it's important for women to understand that sex is more for men than just sex. It's often the only way, and certainly one of the best ways, that they can actually express love and affection.[90]

── 12 ──

The Importance of Communication

"There is nothing more erotic than a good conversation."

~ Author unknown

"Wow! Isn't that beautiful?" You may have said this or heard it said by someone else, about something seen, heard, felt, or smelt. When communicating, all the senses come into play. Oftentimes, you use one or more of those senses and convey your feelings with yet another. We are multifunctional beings when it comes to using our sensory powers!

Rejection

He who is afraid of asking, is ashamed of learning.

~ Danish Proverb

Communicating desire can be difficult. Many times people don't even attempt to ask, for fear of rejection. Sometimes we need to build up courage to ask a question, especially when we fear the answer is going to be negative or even derogatory. There's a modern idiom that describes this situation best as a 'put-down.'

There's nothing worse for a man, when he finally drums up the courage to convey his lustful desires to the object of his passionate feelings, than to feel humiliated. If you're a man, you don't need me to tell you what effect this can have on your libido and your ego.

For women, you and the man can both end up exasperated and frustrated. There's nothing more frustrating than hoping and waiting for this invitation (or a variation thereof), so you can respond positively. When the opportunity never arises, because the man is too shy or ashamed to extend the invitation, it leaves you both out in the cold!

How to Begin?

Used as a slogan by a major telephone company in the UK, the expression '*It's good to talk,* has never been more true. My thesaurus tells me that communication is a noun meaning, among other things—contact, dealings, relations, connection, association, socializing, intercourse, correspondence, dialog, talk, conversation, and discussion.

A little closer to what we're seeking here is the adjective 'communicative,' which means—forthcoming, expansive, expressive, unreserved, uninhibited, vocal outgoing, frank, open, candid, talkative, chatty and loquacious.

This leads to the question—how should we communicate our sexual wants, needs, desires, and hope for acceptance, understanding and reciprocal feelings and actions? The answer is simple. Never be afraid to ask!

True story #1

At a time before the Internet (yes, I am that old!), I had a business acquaintance who worked out of an office on his own in Piccadilly,

London. Knowing he was a randy sort of guy, I asked him what he did with his spare time.

"As you know, Clive," he told me, "London is always buzzing with tourists, particularly in this part. Many of them are really attractive women. During my lunch period, I walk the (sidewalk) outside my office and look out for a pretty girl to take back into the office for sex. When I spot one, I go up to her and say, 'How about a fuck?'"

I was appalled at this crude admission and asked the obvious, "Don't you ever get into trouble?"

To which he replied, "I've had my face slapped a thousand times, but I've had some wonderful fucks!"

Now, I'm not suggesting you follow his example. In fact, I'd be just as appalled today as I was then, but it does illustrate one fact—there are women out there who are just as driven and responsive as a man can be. It's just a case of identifying them and being able to communicate in a way that gets the two people together, without upsetting anyone or being arrested!

True story #2

More recently, I was crossing a road at a major junction in downtown Manhattan. I saw an elegantly dressed, beautiful woman crossing in the opposite direction. She must have noticed my glance of appreciation, because as we passed she asked, "Want to have a good time?"

Clearly I had been approached by a prostitute, but the point I'm making here is it isn't just the vocal approach that gets attention but also the visual—for both parties. And, no, I didn't take her up on her offer!

It is not possible—as some might suggest—to give you the words or expressions to use when talking to the opposite sex. There are no magic words that are guaranteed to get you between the sheets.

I was taught communicating was a two-way affair—question and answer, if you like. However, here on this page, it can only be one-way. We haven't met; therefore, I cannot even guess what you're thinking or what you're hoping to find, other than success. A fair assumption though is you are interested in sex, having sex, having better sex, and doing it with the person you most want to be with.

There are so many variables, some of which may apply to you or just apply to your partner. Whatever you pick up might apply to you today, but I hope it will also prepare you for all your tomorrows. There are those who can express their desires, and then there are those who find it very difficult. Both look to the written word, for answers to their hidden agenda, and this is where I hope you will find a way through these pages.

True story #3

I had been out with a young lady a number of times, and I found her company put a spring in my step, as the saying goes. We were dining out in a London restaurant one evening, and I was looking into the eyes of this lovely girl across the table. Suddenly, I realized I wanted her to be by my side for the rest of my life. I didn't think it would be fair to come right out with a proposal of marriage there and then. I didn't even have a ring to give her, so I began to say, "You're just the sort of girl . . . ." My voice trailed off, because she placed a finger across my lips saying silently, "Not here; not now."

My reason for recalling this story is because this lovely lady—yes, we did get married a year later and, yes, we are still together—not only gave herself the time she needed to consider the proposal but had anticipated what I was about to say, by reading all the signs through eye contact and body language. To be fair, she had already worked out I was an old romantic (still am) and could therefore spot the signals ahead of time.

If you're a male, youth brings you the energy, the drive and the ambition to capture her heart and get her into bed, as soon as she will let you. If you are female, you want him to hold off while you assess his suitability—to care for you, be a good provider, be emotionally strong, and be a perfect father to your children.

'I think the key to any healthy relationship is communication. As with all things intimate, discussing preferences with your partner, in a respectful and caring manner, is critical.'

~ Kimberly Wylie

Very true. However, for many, it's easier said than done.

The first thing to remember is we have one mouth but *two* ears. This is a good way to remind ourselves of the importance of being a good listener. We also have two eyes. Listen and watch; body language can speak volumes. From turning away to placing a hand on your thigh, and all the minor movements in between, keep your eyes open. Don't stare, but eye contact coupled with a growing smile and even a tilt of the head to suggest a little shyness, can convey much of what you find difficult to put into words. 'Are you thinking what I'm thinking?' is a good test to find common ground.

Euphemisms

There are occasions when using direct language is not appropriate, especially when in mixed company. Vulgarity might have its place, even adding spice when used as dirty talk leading up to and during sex. However, there are times when you really do find it difficult to make a suggestion by using proper nouns and adjectives, to convey your message. "Can I insert my penis into your vagina, while I suck your nipples?" doesn't sound half as romantic as, "Shall we make love."

Of course, even euphemisms can be found inappropriate. Consider carefully before asking, 'How about a fuck/shag?" Always think before speaking.

True story #4

My wife and I were on vacation in England's West Country with a couple of old friends. We were watching some sea birds standing on a rocky outcrop of the river entrance, spreading their wings to catch the evening sun. These large and very black birds are Cormorants. Later that evening, having dined and enjoyed each other's company, the four of us stood looking through the window overlooking the river.

"Oh, look," our female friend said pointing to a black seabird busy fishing in the water. "There's a Cormorant."

"That's not a Cormorant," her husband said knowingly. "That's a Shag." (Shags look like Cormorants but are about half the size).

Time came to go to bed. "Come on," our female friend said to her husband, "I fancy a Cormorant."

Humor

Friends often tell my wife and I we're always laughing. Not exactly true. However, we do know that it is our sense of humor that has helped build the unbreakable bond we have forged.

As with all things in life, there is always room for humor in the bedroom. Of course a sigh, a grunt, a moan, a loving word, and even an occasional shout are all well-placed; however, laughter can be appropriate too. If you're having good, carefree, fun sex, enjoy it! Smile! Laugh! Giggle! As long as you're not laughing at your partner or what they are doing, don't be afraid to have fun during sex. Sex doesn't always have to be a serious endeavor of passion. It can be silly sometimes too!

Try to spot the funny side of life and joke about things both in and out of the bedroom. Coupled with body language, a knowing look and a gentle kiss, humor can lubricate the path to the sex. Make her smile. Make him smile. Feel the warmth of togetherness a smile can bring. Hold her hands, kiss her fingertips, breathe gently into her ear, nibble the lobe, and kiss the nape of her neck. If she's tickled by these actions, let her laugh. If you're the girl and you're warmed by these actions, let him know by holding him closer.

Make light of things not going to plan or the way you had wished. Trying new positions or new places sometimes get awkward. A chuckle in recognition when new things aren't working out followed by, "Let's try something/somewhere else." will likely be similar to what was going through your partner's mind, too.

Don't dismiss the old-fashioned missionary position as 'old hat' or for those without imagination. I'll tell you why the missionary position is actually very popular. It's because you can kiss and look at each other—embracing the deepest kind of communication!

Choose the Moment

No good trying to get into deep thought while your partner is involved in another activity that requires concentration—like cooking, driving or picking up a phone call/message. When we first fall in love, we never stop talking. We have real communication. You want to discover how your partner thinks, what they hate and desire, their ambitions, and their limitations. We want to share it all. As our lives progress though, our chats are more likely to be about bills, housekeeping and the kids' schooling.

If you want to know how easily love can fade, get an empty glass jar and every time your partner says, "I love you" put a bean in it. When the jar is full make a note of how long it took to fill. After that, every time your partner says, "I love you" take a bean out of the jar. When the last bean is removed from the jar take a look at the calendar. You'll likely discover it takes much longer to empty as it does to fill. Let's try to do something to put that right—keep up the intimate conversations!

Be honest and kind. Psychologists note it takes five kind words to undo the damage caused by one angry one.

Always be there for each other. Listen, even when it's your turn to talk keep listening (*two* ears, remember?). If you are at the same place as your partner—and I mean a true and declared understanding—your relationship can be indestructible.

Intimate conversations are good—even arousing—but there are good times and not so good times to start such conversations. Devote time to building trust; communicate respect then lead each other into speaking openly about how you like to be touched or even seduced. We all fantasize from time to time. Share your fantasies and be brave about declaring to each other what you like to do, even talking about things you have never done but quite like the idea of trying out.

However, as you lie naked together and are about to have sex, this is *not* the time to ask what she likes in bed. Her mind, and yours, should be totally vacant—not having to think about what to do or what not to do. Sex becomes a purely mechanical adventure (at best) rather than an emotional connection of two minds, allowing them to drift into a blissful union.

Likewise, immediately following sex is not the time for analyzing the act either. "How was it for you?" is a joke. Wait until the next time you're alone with each other and the conversation gets onto your favorite topic.

Security

We all feel insecure from time to time, and little things—actions as well as words—can remove those unsettling moments. From simple gestures, like opening a door or making the coffee to flowers or a surprise date, these actions tell us we are cared for, understood and loved! They make us feel secure. Strive to make your partner always feel secure in how much you love them through both your words and your actions.

Anxiety

Let's get something straight before we take this any further. Guys and gals have the same perplexing degrees of anxiety when it comes to sexual performance. Yes, the guy wants his girl to believe he really knows what he's doing, and the girl wants her guy to feel she had the best sex ever. Remember we talked briefly about women faking orgasm?

A woman will typically only fake an orgasm if she has no chance of getting there with what the man is doing or how he is doing it. One of the primary reasons she fakes it is so she doesn't upset him, to avoid hurting his ego and to end that which is going nowhere.

The woman is also afraid of being judged—just as much as the man is afraid of being judged. She worries about her attractiveness, her desirability, her hair, her breasts, her bottom, her tummy, and her legs. "Will he love me for who I am?" "How will I compare with other women he's slept with?" "What will he expect me to do; will he be caring?"

He worries about his performance. "Will I be able to satisfy her; bring her to orgasm?" "Will I be able to hold off long enough to avoid premature ejaculation?" "Will she think my penis isn't big enough?"

All of the above can typically be applied to youthful singles. By the time you've settled down into a long-term partnership, much of this has been sorted out. However, we still may have concerns that cause anxiety when it comes to our bodies and our sexual performance, even when we've been with a partner for awhile.

The Power of Anticipation

Spontaneous sex is great, but who, with a houseful of kids, TVs and computer screens glaring messages to you and cellphones ringing, can even dream of the opportunity of discarding clothes and having passionate sex in the doorway? Don't give up on spontaneity! With a little careful thought, this can be done.

You might have heard of someone being 'on a promise.' This simply means a partnership has recognized and identified all their environmental situations getting in the way of enjoying sex together and have thought of a way to resolve the problem. You both agree to have sex at a preappointed date and time.

Even if your situation doesn't require such planning ahead, sowing the seed of an idea in the mind of your partner and giving her—or him—time to dwell on the prospect will result in a passion that has been given time to build in the mind. It has often been said the brain is the biggest sex organ, and this anticipation can produce more powerful sex than spontaneous sex. Simply put, this is the power of anticipation. However, if you can be spontaneous, a 'quickie' can lead to something that lasts longer.

There has to be a place and a time you can set aside to enjoy each other. Even if it means locking the bedroom door and waking an hour earlier, many couples discover sex first thing in the day, after a restful night's sleep, is better for them. If it really is impossible to arrange this at home, get a baby sitter and book a room in a hotel. The message here is never give up! Use it or lose it is a strong reminder of what's at stake.

Pillow Talk

Pillow talk, talking and cuddling with your partner after sex, has been found to have significant benefits, according to University of Michigan researcher Dr. Daniel Kruger. In the study he co-authored, Dr. Kruger and his colleagues surveyed 456 volunteers about their sleep patterns and their desire for affection, bonding and communication. The study found that men, in general, fell asleep before their female partners. However, this can be damaging to the relationship.[91]

As Dr. Kruger notes, "(Pillow talk after sex) is the time when couples make promises and establish commitment. The time couples spend together after sex might be as important as what happens before in terms of building a relationship, yet it has rarely been studied."[92]

Other studies share the same results but with some anecdotal differences. Some men admit to trying to exploit their partner's mellow mood following sex, by asking her for a favor. Long-term or short-term, women still want to be intimate. Women are more likely to want to kiss, cuddle and to profess their love after sex. There is, however, one thing both sexes agree on—the importance of saying "I love you" in a committed relationship.

Sexting

Relationship counselors tell me men often prefer typing to talking. They like to use email or instant messaging, as they find it easier to open up. This fact is reflected in the increased use of sexting—sexual text message. Cell phones now give you the means of sending a message anytime and anywhere. It also gives you time to think before you 'speak' or send a message.

For some, overt sexual messages are not nearly as nice or may not be as acceptable as a gentle suggestion. "Just thinking about you is making my heart beat faster." may sound cheesy but will have a far greater impact of acceptability and anticipation, for some people, than, "I wanna fuck you." Of course, if your partner likes it a little naughtier, then perhaps the latter is better. The point is—your message should be geared toward what your partner desires.

A sexting conversation might begin as, "I want you. Now. Here. Hard. Fast." if you are already that close in your relationship. It will likely generate a response, like asking what you intend to do specifically.

Of course, if you're unsure of what your partner will like, it's better to be soft with your approaches, especially with a new relationship. Build trust and respect with, "Would love to take you out to dinner—will tonight be ok?' If you get a positive reply, you might venture a little further with, "Wear something sexy—you look fabulous."

Be Careful with Technology

Nearly everyone has a camera phone nowadays. It is all too easy to upload pictures of yourself and your partner onto social media sites such as Twitter and Facebook. Frequently, these start off as an enthusiastic declaration of a new relationship. Although harmless shots of you and your new significant other will likely be accepted enthusiastically by your friends and family, never post anything racy. Once you post something online, it is there forever, even if you delete the file. You can't unring that Internet bell. A good rule of thumb—is it a picture your grandmother would be OK with displaying in her home? If not, simply don't post it.

Even sending intimate photos privately can be a bad idea. You may think texting or e-mailing your partner a racy picture is a good idea. However, what happens if the two of you break up and your ex is angry with you? They could post that private picture publicly, for the world to see. Even if you're still happily together, if your partner accesses their e—mail on a work computer or uses a company-owned cellphone and receives a racy text, this could even be cause for firing. Many companies have a no tolerance policy when it comes to pornography in the workplace.

A survey of 1,500 men and 1,500 women, aged 16 to 86, was commissioned for the launch of Elizabeth Noble's novel, *The Way We Were*. Noble's novel is the story of childhood sweethearts who reappear in each other's lives years later. Professor Alexander Gordon, a chartered psychologist and member of the British Psychological Society, said the gender difference was 'stark.' He said men tended to tick more superficial boxes, such as looks, to help them decide whether they were 'in love.' Women were a little more complicated and likely to weigh up the pros and cons, before settling on their choice.[93]

"Women are better at reading social situations and are more likely to ask more questions of themselves after meeting someone, like—Is he going to make me feel secure and will he be a good father to my children?" Gordon said. "They are cannier than men at making a lifetime choice."[94]

A Final True Story

My wife and I had just finished a busy day. My wife, had cooked the evening meal, and, as usual, it was lovely. I wrote a note saying, "I think you're fantastic. I love you. XXX" and left it on the kitchen countertop. I was upstairs when I heard her laughing, and I knew she had found the note.

Such a simple communication can truly make your partner feel loved and cherished. Never take your partner for granted. You can never say "I love you" too much.

—— 13 ——

It Started with a Kiss

It started with a kiss

~Hot Chocolate, 1982

Trust scientists to come up with an explanation for even the simplest pleasures!

Helen Fisher, an anthropologist at Rutgers University, tells us that according to a new study, men prefer sloppier, more open-mouthed kissing because saliva contains testosterone, which increases sex drive. She notes, "This suggests they are unconsciously trying to transfer testosterone to turn women on more."[95] Here I was thinking I was just loving those big, wet kisses!

Of course, there are other opinions on kissing. Humans kiss to boost immunity, say University of Leeds researchers, in the UK. Kissing exposes a woman to small doses of cytomegalorivus. Over time, she becomes inoculated against this virus, which is responsible for some problems in pregnancy.[96]

My favorite scientific reasoning for kissing is the anti-depressant effect. Couples who kiss and cuddle a lot are eight times less likely to get depressed than those who do it only during sex.[97]

To speed things up a little in the bedroom, researchers at Lafayette College in the US, tell us to kiss for at least three minutes to boost desire. Kissing reduces levels of the stress hormone cortisol, speeding up the time it takes to be turned on.[98]

Treat it like Dancing

Rowan Pelling, author and Life-Style sex columnist for the Daily Mail in the UK, was asked what was the secret of good kissing. She replied, "Treat it like dancing and follow your partner."[99] This is excellent advice, but she went on to describe various scenarios depicted by friends and correspondents.

Pelling notes there are etiquette concerns that come with kissing. Timing and depth of the tongue probe being two of the most important. Of course, oral hygiene is also a factor. Although our taste and smell can be altered with teeth brushing, mouthwash and gum, there is still a unique taste to each person's mouth. We are genetically programmed to prefer the taste and smell of partners who will be a good reproductive fit for us.[100]

The Perfect Fit

There is also the issue of 'fit',' according to Pelling. As I'm sure you can relate, some mouths just seem to fit our own better. In fact, she notes that mismatched mouths can be the reason why first-time partners feel one or the other is a bad kisser. She even relates a story when she was younger, in which one friend had described a local hunk as 'the perfect kisser.' However, her personal experience was quite the opposite—'saliva-filled disasters' was how she deemed them.[101]

This led to an impromptu survey of a dozen of Pelling's girlfriends, regarding what they felt was the perfect kiss. Where some preferred the more chaste but passionate kisses found in classic movies, others liked soft butterfly kisses along the edges of the mouths, and still others wanted tongues that explore, embrace and rehearse for the sex to come.[102] Clearly, even when it comes to kissing, we're all different!

Of course, don't forget areas other than the mouth. Nibbles and kisses on the neck and ears can drive your partner wild. Try their eyelids, their shoulders, even kisses to the forehead can make your partner feel cherished. The important thing here is to find out what your partner likes. Follow your partner's lead.

With a new partner, start off slowly. Pay attention to the pressure, speed and depth of the kiss. Rarely will a woman appreciate you shoving your tongue down her throat right off the bat, without a clear invitation to do so. If you want to move things to the next level, gently lead into it and see if your partner is willing to follow. "Men turned out to have equally strong opinions on the subject, and one doctor friend confessed to a fear of 'aggressive kissers,'" according to Pelling.[103]

Prepare for the Kiss

Preparing to kiss just makes good sense. The last thing you want is to have an eager kissing partner, and you worried about your breath. Preparation begins with regular brushing and flossing. Little bits of food trapped between your teeth can really cause oral odor and taste issues. If your date includes dinner, bring a disposable toothbrush with you and excuse yourself to the restroom after you eat. You'll feel that much more confident if it comes to a goodnight kiss.

Smokers are a particularly difficult issue. Unless your partner is also a smoker, chances are your partner will still notice a slight odor/taste, even if you've recently brushed your teeth. Fresh gum or mints can help mask that smell, but quitting smoking is an even better solution! It's healthier for your body, your sex life and makes it much more enjoyable to kiss you!

Oral preparation, as Pelling notes, also involves the dentist. "Regular trips to the dentist are important, too—much of the worst halitosis is caused by tooth decay and gum disease. I know a number of attractive people, of both sexes, who repel suitors because of their dragon's breath."[104]

—— 14 ——

More About Foreplay

I think you're running into a lot of trouble
if your idea of foreplay is,
'Brace yourself honey, here I come!'

~ Phil McGraw

By definition 'foreplay' precedes the 'main event.' Although after talking about the subject of foreplay with friends, I found many people had differing opinions on the subject. Most people immediately think about techniques—places to touch, places to kiss, and places to caress. However, for some, foreplay begins with a look, a smile, a sound (musical or natural, such as the sound of surf), or a visual reminder of a romantic moment previously enjoyed that led to the main event.

I titled this chapter *MORE About Foreplay* because foreplay is to be found everywhere in this book. Many believe a man needs very little foreplay to achieve an erection, which is often considered to be the goal of foreplay for men, and that a woman's needs require more attention to foreplay, in order to be ready for full coital sex.

Neither of these statements is necessarily true and certainly is not applicable to every man and woman. It would be correct to say an erect penis is required for penetrative sex and equally true that a lubricated vagina, which can be achieved naturally or with spittle or bottled lube, is all that is required for the penis to enter. However, where's the joy, the love, the sharing of warmth and emotional ties in that though? This is why foreplay is important. Without foreplay, you are not making love—you're just fucking.

Kissing and Cuddling

Foreplay can begin with a conversation, perhaps over dinner. There are countless triggers to open the door to foreplay. The aroma of a warm body, a particular perfume, the briefest of touches, even movement (like the way your partner dances or even holds a glass) are all things that can arouse your senses and thoughts of intimacy. Whatever the trigger, the most practiced and prevalent action leading to foreplay is simply kissing and cuddling.

The Importance of Foreplay

What does foreplay do for you, and why is it so important?

The case for foreplay for women is well documented. What man has not heard or read about women needing to be 'in the mood?' This is a simplified and slightly misleading expression of a woman's physical and emotional needs, which she yearns for, so she can do what she wants to do freely and totally.

Empty her mind of the mundane household and work thoughts and replace them with the erotic desires prompted by the closeness of the man she loves—his strength, his control, his confidence. During foreplay, blood flow to her genitals and breasts increases, her sexual sensory nerve endings become more exposed and the lubricating glands in her vagina and around her vulva begin to excrete.

The time it takes for this to happen will vary from woman to woman and from partner to partner. Other factors that affect the time it will take include the opportunity and location and the influence of external factors, such as the risk of interruption. Definitely make sure the kids are asleep and the television is turned off!

Foreplay For Men

I have been unable to find anything written about men's foreplay needs. Of course, he only has himself to blame for this, by making a joke of the whole situation and concentrating on ensuring his woman is happy. Guys, you need to know the girls in your life are every bit as turned on by sharing and feeling your passion build as you are of theirs!

Benefits for the Man

The benefits of foreplay to a man have to be experienced to be believed. This is probably why the older and more experienced man takes his time. It's as much for his own enjoyment as for his partner's. It's true the first indication of arousal is his erection, but that really is only the beginning. This is not to say there will be moments when you are both so ready little or no foreplay is required. For times like this, surprise her with a quickie.

When you jump her out of the blue, it makes her feel like she's so irresistible you simply can't wait to have her. Right when she gets home, pull her in for a deep kiss to get her going. Relieve her of any bags she's carrying and lead her to the couch, bed or kitchen table, where you will have already stashed a bottle of lube nearby. Don't totally undress her; just lift up her skirt or pull down her pants. Then use your lubed fingers to massage her clitoris while whispering how hot she is in her ear. The more aroused you are, the faster she'll get into it. (Of course, there will be times when she's not game. If this happens, let it go and try another night.)

Before I go any further, I can hear you asking, "What happens to a man's arousal during foreplay?"

Many women think all they need to concentrate on for foreplay and her man is his penis. It's true this will produce a male orgasm or ejaculation. If you're in a hurry, then that's all you have to do. Indeed, there is a parallel here with women. Masturbating, whether by yourself or by your partner, produces a satisfactory result but absolutely nothing like the results of full sex preceded by plenty of foreplay.

Male Foreplay Erogenous Zones

There are many sensitive places around a man's body, and it can be fun discovering what your man likes best. Babs says,

> *Don't forget men have nipples, too. Foreplay should include his nipples in your list of his sensitive spots. Some men are less sensitive in this area than others. Some like it rough; some like it gentle. Find out what he likes best, and you'll discover the more often they get a treat, the more sensitive they become—just like ours!*

Each man will have his own preferences and the journey toward the ultimate goal can, and should, be as enjoyable for him as it is for her. For many, foreplay will be considered a major tease; this is not far from the truth. The idea is to discover what places you can feel or stroke, lick or kiss, that brings him close to orgasm without actually cumming. What can you do to keep him in that state?

This is where established relationships benefit most. The woman knows exactly how far she can go with her man, having learned over the years how to recognize the signs he makes—voluntary or involuntary.

Something to Try With Your Man

While on his back, have your guy spread his legs and raise his knees so you have easy access to his perineum and anus. Tease him and build his anticipation by:

- First run the palm of your hand along the underside of his upper thighs, not quite touching but close enough to tickle the hairs on his legs in those places.

- Follow this by pressing a finger firmly against the perineum, the point half-way between the base of his scrotum and his anus, and rotate your finger in little circles.

- He may encourage you to move your finger closer and even into his anus.

- A single finger circling his anus can be a tremendous stimulant.

A point worth noting here is men are very similar to women in one respect. Many don't think how stimulation in two different spots at the same time heightens the pleasure of orgasm.

Overdrive

During this part of foreplay, the man's prostate gland goes into overdrive to top-off his seminal sack. His Cowper's gland oozes clear lube along the urethra to slick the passage of seminal fluid at the point of ejaculation. The blood vessels dilate maximizing his erection. Just before ejaculation, there's an involuntary raising of the scrotum closer to the body, to protect the testes when excited.

You can imagine what all this activity can bring to his point of orgasm. The longer you can hold him close to the point of no return without allowing him to spill over into ejaculation, the greater the impact of his orgasm when you or he decides to let his ejaculate fly.

Ideas to Put Your Man into Overdrive

Following are just a few ideas to really put your man into overdrive:

- **Mirrors**—Although you may not want to permanently affix mirrors on your ceiling, there is something undeniably sexy about seeing you and your lover in a mirror reflection. With this in mind, give him a hand-held mirror to use, so he can get a better view of you going down on him, or position yourselves so you have sex doggy-style, you can both watch yourselves in the mirror above your dresser.

- **Private Peep Show**—If your guy is into it, masturbate in front of him. Some guys find the site of a woman pleasuring herself very erotic.

- **Be a Tease**—Don't be afraid to tease him a little bit. Kiss your way down his stomach, getting oh-so-close to his penis, and then move back up again, smiling wickedly up at him. When you do finally give him the attention he's longing for, it'll be just that much sweeter.

- **Lavish Attention on His Penis**—Most men enjoy oral sex. That's not an issue. However, there is something even more amazing when a woman completely lavishes attention on a penis. Don't just immediately go for the traditional blow job. Run your tongue, in a broad lick, along the shaft of his penis. Swirl your tongue around the glans. Kiss the tip lovingly, looking up into his eyes, letting him know how much you cherish every bit of him.

- **Use Both Hands**—When stroking the shaft of his penis, with a little lube on your hand, also gently caress his glans, giving him double the sensation.

Communication and Foreplay

It has been said—sex improves communication. I will argue also—communication improves sex. It certainly improves the pathway to sex!

Foreplay can begin with the question, "Shall we make love?" or a statement, "Let's make love." Even this will have been preceded by circumstances and environment that quicken the pulses and give you the courage to express your desire for intimacy. You might text each other with racy, one-word messages during the work-day to increase the anticipation of what you can look forward to that night.

As we talked about in Chapter 12, the key is communication!

Now It's Her Turn

Although it may be a bit stereotypical, don't fail to spend time on foreplay for your woman. Although sometimes she'll be in the mood right away, other times she may need a bit more coaxing. Be patient, and don't rush her. Listen to the signs her body is giving you, from the soft moans and heavy breathing to the way she angles her body, encouraging more contact with whatever you're doing.

The neck is a super-sensitive area and a great way to begin to drive her wild, especially the area between her ear and her collarbone. Because the skin is thinner here, it's more sensitive than other areas of the neck. Kiss, suck and nibble this area gently. Or, lick her lightly then blow your breath across the area. The warmth of your tongue contrasted with the coolness of your breath against the area you just licked will likely make her shiver with pleasure.

At the bottom of the neck, the skin is a little bit thicker. This means it can take a little more pressure, especially where the neck joins with the shoulder. You can be a little more aggressive here, but again, listen to her words and/or her body language to discover what she really likes.

Ideas to Put Your Woman in Overdrive

Try these ideas, to really add some heat in the bedroom, for your woman.

- Challenge yourself to kiss and touch areas that you don't normally think of during foreplay. Behind the knees, the back of the neck, and even the wrists can all be very sensitive areas, when caressed or kissed gently.

- During oral sex, draw a figure eight with your tongue over her clitoris, so it hits it from every angle.

- During oral sex, don't forget you still have fingers to excite her too. Insert a finger into her vagina and stroke her G-spot with a come-hither motion.

- Position yourself perpendicular to her body, so your tongue can move across her clitoris, rather than up and down, for an even more intense sensation.

— 15 —

Making Love: A Woman's & A Man's Perspective

A loving heart is the beginning of all knowledge.

~ Thomas Carlyle

Love Matters

My choice of words is deliberate. 'Making love' may be considered old-fashioned; however, in my opinion, this phrase is a better description than simply the term 'sex.'

Sex is a broad description of what animals do. Yes, that does include humans, but it's an act with the singular purpose to procreate.

Unlike animals, humans have developed a higher sense of purpose when it comes to sex. It's an emotional sense, and a sense that urges us to be with, and look after, our chosen partner. For an all-encompassing description, we call it 'love.'

My reasons for reminding you of the obvious are two people in love with each other and having sex allows both exploring and enjoying each others' bodies, to levels not available to those having casual sex just for the sake of it. I wanted to make this point so as not to mislead you into thinking love and sex are the same things. In this chapter, you will read about the detailed practicalities of enjoying sex. If two people are in love with each other, the techniques will heighten what is described.

With the sophisticated knowledge humans have, we have a further advantage over animals—the use of contraceptive methods! We can choose whether we wish to protect against pregnancy or not. Sex, therefore, becomes recreational. We hone our skills and look forward to frequent and amazing sex!

A Woman's Perspective

What Does it Feel Like?

While I was following a forum (PEGym.com), the question came up—"What does it feel like for a woman, when a guy cums inside her?"

The answers are not only interesting, they also reinforce my point about the added benefit love brings. Katie, a forum member, replied,

> *I love it when my boyfriend cums inside of me. I sometimes can feel the pulsing in his penis right before he is ejaculating, but I can't feel the actual semen. The physical aspects of this don't make me feel anything special, but the emotional does.*

> *With other guys that I have had casual sex with, or that I didn't feel anything for, it didn't matter to me where they would cum. However, I love my boyfriend, and when he cums inside of me it feels very right. I feel close to him. I like being that close to him when he cums, especially if I can see his face and hold his body at the same time and feel how his whole body reacts to the orgasm. It sort of feels like I'm more a part of his orgasm if he cums inside of me."*

At this point, Batwoman joined in:

The emotional part is huge—that is the biggest part (most of the time) of what I feel when a man cums inside me. How good that part is depends completely on the relationship. For a woman, feeling a man you love and desire cum deep inside you is a marvelous experience. It can be a heart-pounding thrill. However, if he is a casual partner or someone you don't care much about, it is less good.

In terms of what us females feel physically, it can be quite limited. You need to remember that the vagina does not have a lot of sensory nerves inside—far fewer than regular skin has. What we feel also varies according to how aroused and tight we are. Sometimes I feel more than other times. The best is when I am very aroused but have had an orgasm recently, so I am nice and wet and tight all at the same time. Then I can really feel him best.

As to exactly what I feel vaginally, when he cums . . . it is the spasming and pulsing of his cock that I can feel. There is no sensation associated with the release of fluids other than the feel of his cock pumping.

The rest of what is going on also affects what I experience too, of course—what parts of his body are pressed against mine, what position we are in, whether or not I have my arms or legs around him, and so on. I had not thought about it before, but it might be that it is easier to feel a man's cock pulsing when he is not pressed in as deep as he can go. I am not sure about that.

When I know he is getting close to cumming, I tend to key in on his breathing (which can tell me a lot about what he is feeling) and his eyes (if I can see them) because that increases the feeling of connection. Emotional and physical sensations tend to blur together then. Sometimes his orgasm is so intense for him that it almost washes over me too. Not physically exactly, but in some strange intermediate between the physical and emotional. That is very exotic and exciting."

Not Missing the Big O

My wife and I are very close friends with another couple—Roly and Babs. We were talking about orgasms and how frequently, or infrequently, the girls achieved an orgasm. Babs argued men seemed to think they've failed if they reached the orgasmic state, but their partners didn't.

"You don't have to go for gold every single time," she said. "There are occasions when I don't feel it necessary, but that doesn't mean I'm not enjoying it. Some of the best sex I've ever had didn't result in an orgasm for me."

Batwoman agrees with Babs:

> *It can be about timing, Sometimes I really feel like sex but an orgasm does not feel particularly necessary or attainable. That may be hard for a guy to understand, but it's true. In my case, if we've had a lot of sex lately, and I've already had a few orgasms in the last 24 hours, I may not be able to easily get to the peak of arousal that's necessary for me to cum. That does not mean that I can't get most of the way up the mountain and really enjoy being there. Sustained arousal can feel fabulous, even if it never quite gets to the peak. If I've cum recently, staying on that plateau maybe where I prefer to be, rather than struggling to try to cum again, since it is really more enjoyable.*

A Man's Perspective

*There is a road from the eye to the heart that
does not go through the intellect.*

~ Gilbert K. Chesterton

There are two major factors influencing a man's perspective—
testosterone and fear. A third factor quickly follows when a man has
fallen in love—a need to please.

A man doesn't want to talk about sex; he just wants to get down to
it. If the subject ever comes up, when he's casually talking to friends,
he will always feign 'no problem in that department,' even if he is a
complete failure in his own eyes.

A guy has been equipped with a Ferrari between his legs. This
wasn't his choice; he was born with it. He needs to learn how to use
and control it. If he's lucky, he will find a woman that will show him
the way to please her. Until this happens, he is expected to behave
like a gentleman—often having to hide the fact that he has an erection
in his pants and what feels like several pints of semen just dying to
get out.

The Early Days of Manhood

The early days of manhood set the tone of confusion and
frustration for young men. He endures nocturnal emissions
(involuntary ejaculations, AKA 'wet dreams') while asleep and
spontaneous erections prompted by seeing a shapely body. Both
situations prompt deep embarrassment.

His next stage, the time of first 'conquests' (as his joking peers
would say), is swimming in fear. Will it be obvious that he doesn't
have much experience in bed? Will she be pleased? How should he
begin, and what should he do? Is his equipment 'man enough' for
the job? Often, the time comes and so does he. The excitement was

just too much, and the Ferrari sped off like a rocket, which results in more embarrassment.

Of course with time and experience, things start to calm down, and the young man begins to think about his approaches. He appreciates techniques that will bring both himself and his sexual partner closer together, maximizing the enjoyment of sex for them both. With luck, genuine love will follow and make it amazing. Self-doubt diminishes, and his confidence grows.

Most women think that all a man has to do to reach orgasm is stroke his penis, and he will ejaculate. Job done.

In truth, unless just arriving at puberty, there's a whole lot more going on. Touch, sight, smell, warmth, and imagination all play a part in a man's sexual feelings and performance, and not necessarily in that order. There is also hope. Hope that his partner will guide him to her own preferences, so that he can concentrate on satisfying and not just 'holding off' in the hope she will reach an orgasmic state, never mind what he's doing.

If the word 'insecure' springs to mind, that is probably true of all men the first time they find themselves naked with a woman. That feeling vanishes when a man's in love. He becomes secure in the knowledge his partner is on the same plane and their voyage of discovery is going to be mutually enjoyable. The experienced lover will naturally be confident as well.

What Does Sex Feel Like for a Man?

So, what does the sex act feel like for a man? It's a journey shared with another body his hands and fingers touch, his lips brush against and kiss, and his nose detects female scents that arouse his sexual being. The sight of her breasts, her nipples and her pubic mound bring a rush of blood to his penis, which causes an erection. His pulse quickens.

The harder his erection, the fuller a man's groin feels. He senses the build up of semen as it's ready to fly from his body. He knows when equally aroused his partner's body is ready to receive, as his is ready to give.

His breathing becomes shallower. As he gets closer to orgasm, a man feels a sense of detachment that sweeps his mind and his body tenses. Some men will make noises ranging from a whimper to a full-blown howl.

He wants to thrust forward as much as he can, and a series of involuntary contractions deep within his groin rush his semen up and out of his penis. If he remembers, and practices, he can totally relax his entire body immediately before the ejaculation. This produces the effect of sending waves of pleasure from his head to his toes—the equivalent of the female 'whole body orgasm.'

Deeper breathing follows a man's ejaculation, and a warm feeling of togetherness brings with it a desire to hold the position while the half—dozen or so contractions subside, followed by his penis becoming flaccid. It isn't always the same. Sometimes not all the seminal fluid leaves the body, in which case his penis will remain hard, and a second ejaculation encouraged by further stimulation is possible.

Different situations will also produce varying degrees of intensity. This ranges from the simple feeling of release produced by masturbation to heart-thumping, painfully hard erections with high volume ejaculations and multiple contractions—as many as a dozen—produced by extraordinary couplings.

An extreme example, and certainly no ordinary occurrence for any man (unless he has a medical problem), was related to me by Roly:

> *I was a teenager when I had the opportunity to lie naked, alongside a beautiful girl, who was also totally naked. I wanted to show her what it was like when a man*

ejaculated—something she had never witnessed before. I was in an extremely high state of arousal, with an almost painfully hard erection, thanks to being in full view of this lovely girl's body.

It didn't take many strokes of my penis to reach orgasm. However, to my absolute dismay, even though I could feel the strongest of pulsating contractions nothing emerged from my penis.

I was at a loss for words, and I was certain that I had disappointed her. We heard her parents arriving unexpectedly, and she dressed quickly and went down to greet them. She left me and my now permanent erection in the bedroom. I couldn't understand why my penis wouldn't go flaccid, let alone cum. You can imagine the antics I had to go through to make sure my erection wasn't showing through my trousers before I descended the stairs, pretending I had been in the bathroom.

I now know, having learned how strong the PC muscle is, that it is possible to clamp that group of muscles so tightly that not only does it totally restrict blood flow out of the penis, but it can also clamp shut the urethra, which prevents semen from leaving the body. Of course, when it does finally relax, and following the contractions normally associated with ejaculation, all the seminal fluid dribbles free from you penis—the final embarrassment!"

What Roly experienced is known as retrograde ejaculation. The semen is redirected into the bladder and then expelled when you next urinate. In Roly's case, it appears not all of the fluid went into the bladder, which is why he experienced dribbling after the event.

—— 16 ——

Positions and Locations

Accept what life offers you and try to drink from every cup.
All wines should be tasted; some should only be
sipped, but with others, drink the whole bottle.

~ Paulo Coelho

It doesn't take a genius to work out what goes where for sex and the best positions to accomplish the desired result. However, there are ways to make it more enjoyable and places to make it more fun. Plus, there are things we can do to heighten sensations. All of this contributes to keeping our intimacy going and avoids routine and prevents complacency from creeping into our loving relationship with each other. Once complacency sets in, you risk sex becoming dull, uninteresting, boring!

Traditional Positions

Fundamentally, there are really only three positions for coital sex:

- The man lies on top of woman (see Fig.7)

- The woman lies on top of man, or

- The woman is on all fours (doggie) and the man penetrates her from behind.

Figure 7: Missionary Position

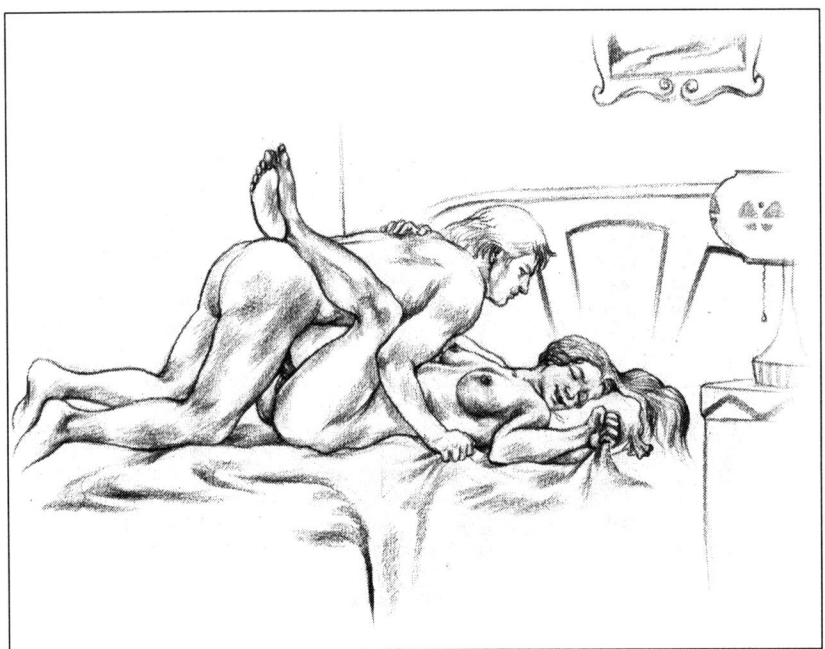

Doggie Style Addition

In doggie-style, the woman can make a downward V with her fingers and place them over her labia, to put pleasuring pressure on the clitoris. This will also add to his pleasure as he feels her fingers down there.

Beyond Traditional

Although missionary, woman-on-top and doggie-style are probably the three most common sexual positions, we're looking for more interesting and exciting ways to enjoy sex!

As we discussed earlier, both men and women have sensory nerve endings that, when given the right treatment, send sexually stimulating signals through our bodies, which leads to orgasm. We understand these areas aren't simply limited to breasts, the vagina and the penis. Now, we need to know the best ways we can take advantage of this knowledge, in the bedroom.

Missionary Alternatives—Man on Top

- **Alternative 1 (Scissors Position)**—For a tighter fit during missionary sex, have the woman bring her legs together and up toward herself, then rest them both on one of the man's shoulders or keep them high and straight. The woman may start with her legs spread, one against each shoulder, then swing one leg over the other, thus forming the 'scissors' position (see Figure 8). Have a pillow handy to raise her bottom and help align entry of his penis, if needed.

- **Alternative 2**—For the woman to get better leverage during missionary sex, have the woman lie with her head toward the foot of the bed and put her feet up against the wall, to use her legs to push back and forth underneath him.

The CAT (Coaxial Alignment Technique)

When asked what he thought to be the #1 position for the best sex, my doctor friend began by reminding us, "It cannot be stressed too much that it is incumbent upon the male to extend the foreplay to the point that the female participant is ready to proceed." Good thought!

The woman should be warmed up and fully aroused. Research has shown it takes a woman approximately ten minutes to become fully aroused.[105] Both partners being fully warmed up should be mandatory, before following any of the positional suggestions.

Figure 8: Missionary Alternative 1 (Scissors Position)

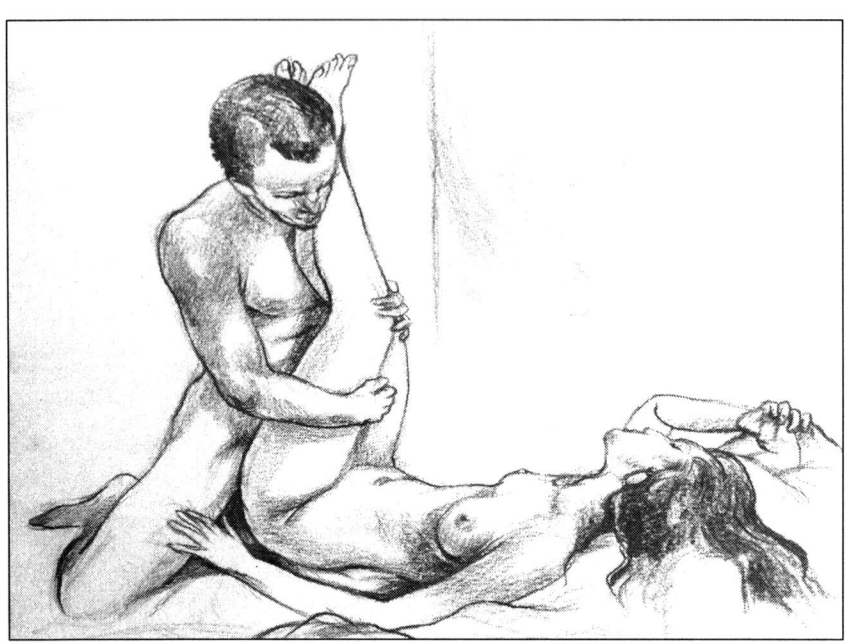

He went on to also remind us,

> *The chief point of stimulation in the female is in the clitoris, and the clitoris points somewhat downwards. For this reason, it makes sense for the male to get the shaft of his penis, after entry (to the vagina), to be perpendicular to the clitoris in order for the entire length of his shaft to rub against the clitoris with each thrust and retraction.*

> *This is best accomplished by inserting the penis all the way, then lifting the male's entire body in a move toward the female's head. This brings the shaft and the clitoris into maximum contact with each other and yields an unimaginable climax. There is no comparison to the more common in-and-out motion that satisfies the male but not always the female.*

The foregoing describes the Coaxial Alignment Technique (CAT), and the Doc strongly recommends it. Incidentally, so do I. As noted above, the CAT is performed in the missionary position, with the woman underneath the man. There's no reason why it shouldn't work with the woman on top; she simply reverses the move so she's in control of when it feels right. Try both ways to discover what is best for you.

There could also be another benefit to using the CAT, the good doctor forgot to mention—it is more than likely that the head of the man's penis will be rubbing along the first couple of inches of the front wall of the woman's vagina. This is the most sensitive part of her vagina and the area where the G-spot can be found. He'll be stimulating that spot as well as the clitoris—an excellent combination!

If the man finds himself unable to stand the heightened sensations any longer and reaches the point of no return, he can resist lowering his body in order to achieve the deepest penetration, which is a natural desire when reaching orgasm, and stay in the CAT position. This will mean his ejaculate will smother the G-spot area, and the woman will feel a 'tingling' or 'tickling' sensation that will only add to her own orgasmic experience or help speed her toward it.

Woman on Top—And in Control

With the woman's legs straightened out along the man's, and using her elbows to take her weight, she guides him in, in the traditional woman—on-top position. She decides the speed and depth of his thrusting penis. She can place her legs outside of his or inside of his, or even one leg between his and the other on the outside. She should observe his reactions and continue appropriately.

There are several advantages for the woman while the man is lying on his back. While the woman is warming up to it (foreplay), she can wrap her fingers around his penis and press it against her labia. She can then rub herself up and down it to get both aroused and prolong the anticipation.

In woman-on-top, as she is sliding up his penis, she should contract her vaginal muscles, squeezing her way up his member. She then releases and slides back down his penis. The clenching of the muscles will help her reach orgasm and give him a tight fit.

Once the woman is straddling him, there are three more positions she can take up.

Cowgirl:

While the woman straddles her guy (see Figure 9), she clenches her legs so his arms and torso are pinned down. As he keeps still, she rolls her hips in a clockwise direction. Switch to counter clockwise, then back every 30 seconds. She can also simply rock her hips back and forth while maintaining clitoral contact with his pubis. The grinding of her clit against his pubis, while his penis is in full penetration, is every bit as good for him as it is for her.

If the woman's hair is really long and she's in woman-on-top position, she can lean back and place both hands on the bed behind her with her head tilted back. He'll get a full view of her breasts and torso and a tickling sensation from the feeling of her hair on his legs.

Reverse Cowgirl:

This is the same as the Cowgirl position, but straddling him so the woman is facing toward his feet, as illustrated in Figure 10. This is a better position for him to reach her posterior A-spot. The same moves as described for Cowgirl apply here. Plus, she can lean forward so her nipples brush his knees. Yes, even men have sensitive knees, and the brushing motion gives an erotic tickling sensation to him as well as allows him a bigger and better view of her anus—another turn-on for many fellas. If the woman enjoys a little anal fingering, she should tell him at this point; his hands are free!

Figure 9: Cowgirl Position

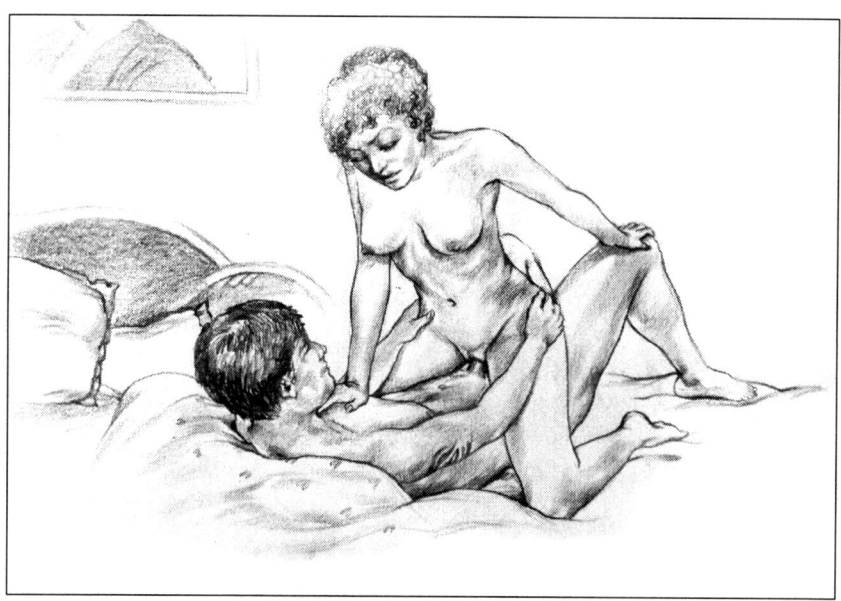

Figure 10: Reverse Cowgirl Position

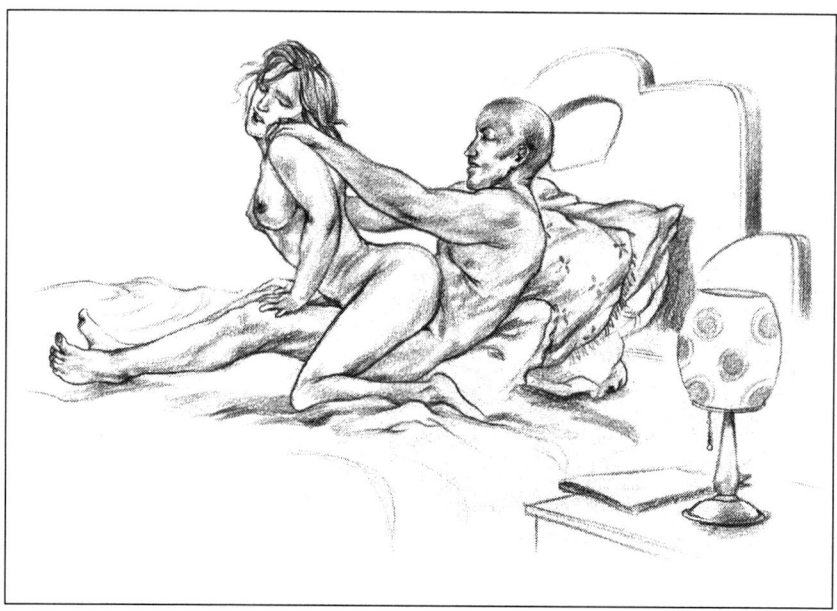

Cross-Legged:

This position is incredibly intimate, as it not only allows you to maintain eye contact, but it puts you nose-to-nose with your partner. The man sits cross-legged on either the floor or bed, and the woman sits on his lap, with her legs wrapped around his back. The woman rocks back-and—forth, grinding her clitoris on his pubis. He can flex his hips upward and increase penetration. Try changing the angle a little, and have the woman lean back slightly,

Figure 11: Cross-Legged Position

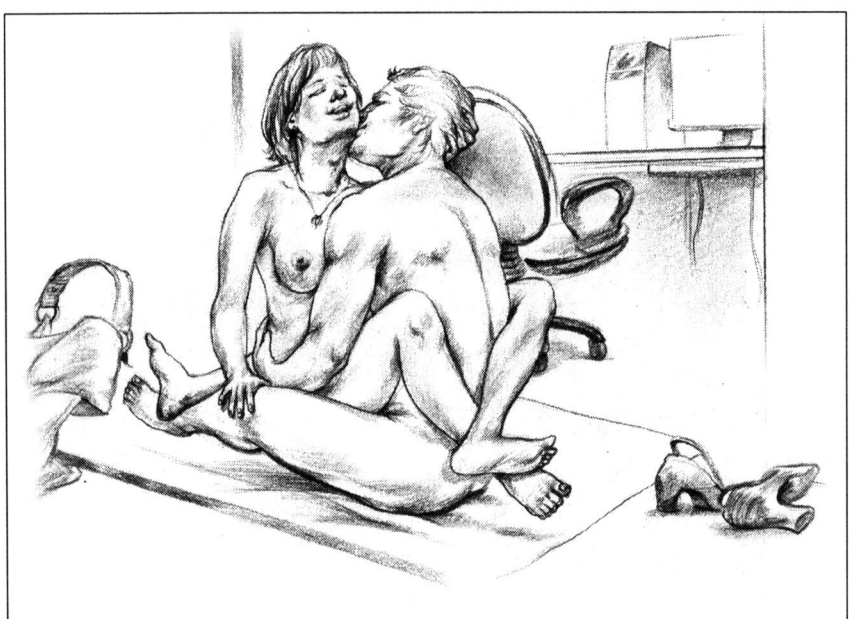

Face Sitting:

There are occasions when you decide it's 'her turn.' By this, I mean an unselfish act carried out on the woman, by her man, for her to enjoy without having to do anything at the time but enjoy the sensations. This is a good prelude to full-on sex.

Don't worry, ladies, this is as much a turn-on for your man as it is a thrill for you. Squat comfortably across his face, as shown in Figure 12, and lean back slightly so your elbows are locked out straight, and your hands are placed on his chest. You can see, from the illustration, how he could place his hands on her thighs and flex his biceps to pull her vulva down onto his mouth.

Figure 12: Face Sitting Position

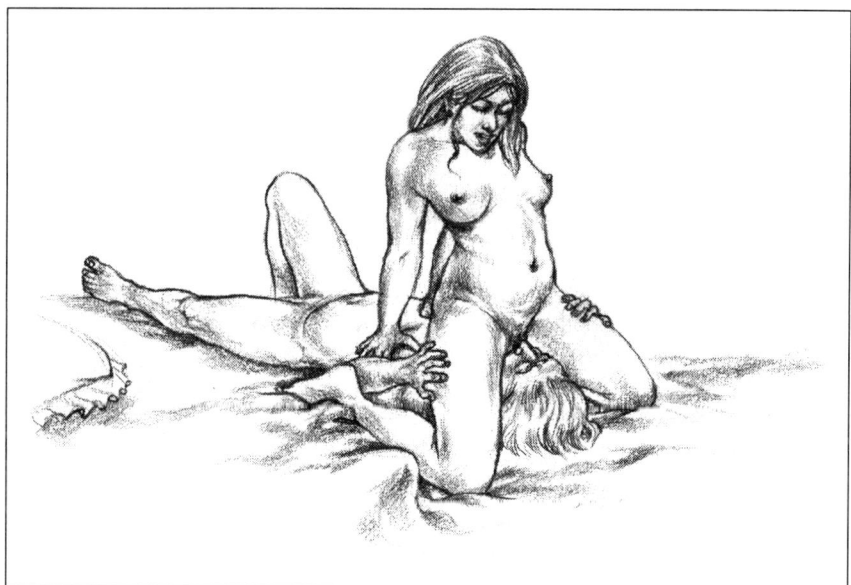

Sixty-Nine:

This oral sex position, shown in Figure 13, can be performed with either the man or the woman on top. One partner lays on their back, while the other kneels over their face, bending forward. Either way, the woman's head is positioned with the man's penis, and the man's head is positioned with the woman's vagina. Whichever partner is on top has the most control. However, the bottom partner does have both of their hands free, to explore other areas of their partner's body or to act as a limiting force to how close their partner can get to their face.

Figure 13: Sixty-Nine Position

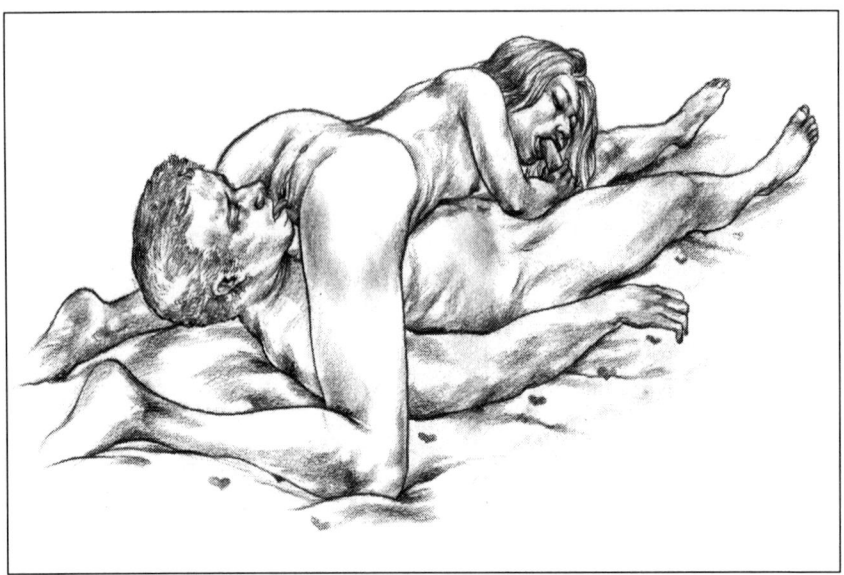

Teasing and Prolonging the Experience

Ladies, have him tease you by varying his thrust technique—entering you with just the tip of his penis and then going only halfway in or stroking you on the outside with his member. He can even swirl inside you, grinding with a circular motion. This can be done in any position that allows penetration.

Slow Down

Gals, as you feel yourself nearing orgasm, slow down to an intensity of about 75 percent of your full speed. Stay there for one minute and then pick up the pace again. This technique will make your orgasm even more intense.

The same goes for the man. Let her know when you feel the orgasm coming on but want it delayed. Stop moving and hold that intimate position for 60 seconds, then slowly pick up the rhythm again. For couples who know each other's signs and keep in eye contact, this can prolong your lovemaking for as long as you both wish.

Batwoman agrees:

> *I like the idea of staying still but inside her. That gives you an intimate moment together that can work other ways for you. Just say, "Baby, I want to slow this down and make it last, stay still . . . ." and kiss her. Look into her eyes, groan, smile, whatever. Keep her part of it; let her know how much she turns you on. Girls love to know they are that good at working you up, and she won't feel rejected if you stay inside her. Just relax, take your time and then pick up the pace again, when you're ready.*

More Ideas to Add Heat to Your Sexual Positions

Here's some more suggestions to add more heat to your sexual positions.

- **Massage His Perineum**—Ladies, you can intensify your guy's orgasm by massaging his perineum. Rub two fingers, in a circular motion, about an inch behind his testicles, for 30 seconds before he orgasms.

- **Sex Challenge**—Challenge yourself and your partner to have sex each day for a month. Having sex more often is like creating a big libido snowball. The more you have it, the more the hormones in your body will make you want it.

- **Sensuous Materials**—There are some materials that feel absolutely sensuous when used during sex. Leather, feathers, velvet, and faux-fur can all be gently stroked along exposed skin to heighten sensations during sex. A beaded necklace, one that does not have exposed string or wire, can be lubed up and played across the shaft of a man's penis or up and down a woman's entire vulva, for a whole new level of arousal.

- **Hair Pulling**—The scalp has thousands of nerve endings. When a woman is aroused, these nerves are on high alert, so hair pulling can be quite erotic. Of course, as with all things sexual, make sure this is something she's into. Always start gently and let her tell you how hard she wants it. Also, never just grab a few strands, but rather grab a generous handful. Further, some women feel like hair pulling in doggie-style is demeaning, while others don't mind at all, and still others are too tender-scalped to enjoy hair pulling. This is where communication is key, because we're all different.

- **Don't Forget the Breasts**—Guys, breasts aren't just for foreplay. Although they are definitely a great tool to get aroused and ready for the main event, don't forget about them once the actual sex starts. Mouths and hands on her breasts can help her reach orgasm more quickly, and make the Big O more explosive when it does come. Additionally, don't just focus on her nipples. Her entire breasts are a great erogenous zone waiting for your attention.

- **Clitoral Stimulation**—It's not uncommon for a woman to only be able to orgasm with clitoral stimulation. For this reason, no matter what position you're in, the man should try rubbing her clitoris, or allow her to do so herself. Every woman prefers to be stimulated in different ways. In fact, she could prefer something different on different days, depending on her mood. However, a good rule of thumb is to start off softly and slowly, building up speed and pressure.

- **Kissing**—Most guys stop kissing once foreplay is over and full intercourse begins. That's a shame. Kissing not only will make your partner feel more connected to you emotionally, allowing her to open up and relax. Kissing will also keep the arousal at its peak for both of you, whether it's slow, deep romantic kisses, or kisses that are hungry and fervent.

Speaking personally, I find the orgasmic impact is multiplied if we are connected at both ends—penis deep in the vagina and tongues deep in each other's mouths. If we have been motoring along just enjoying the intimacy but my wife decides she wants to orgasm, she plants her mouth hard against mine and dives in with her tongue. She knows this simple move excites me so much it takes me to the next level, the point of no return, and I can reach orgasm within seconds. There is a certain magic, and it is decidedly satisfying when we cum together.

Be Aggressive

There's a reason why Fifty Shades of Grey has been a break-away hit in the world of fiction. One thing women often complain about is their partner simply isn't aggressive enough. Now, we're not talking about negative aggression, but rather a man who takes charge with utter confidence in his sexual prowess. Guys, even if you're not that confident, acting like you are can be incredibly erotic for your partner. Here are a few things you can try, to give the feeling you're in control.

- While in the missionary position, capture her wrists in one of your hands, and hold them above her head.

- In the cowgirl position, firmly hold on to her hips and guide her movements.

- Change positions with authority. If she's on top, and you want to switch to missionary, do it firmly and quickly. Don't be timid about it.

Locations

During the early years of our marriage, my wife and I moved a few times. Each new home presented us with the opportunity to discover new places to make love. I imagine it must be a little like the animal 'nesting' principle.

The bedroom is an obvious starting place, but not necessarily the most erotic. The living and dining areas all provide different aspects and advantages. It would bring humor into our sexual adventures when facing the challenges presented by having sex on the stairs, in hallways and the smallest room. The kitchen table and being surrounded by all that food gives an added frisson of excitement to the occasion. Even door frames can be utilized, as described previously by a Cosmopolitan reader. Open spaces provide a thrill. This is probably because of the danger element and anticipating being caught in the act.

One piece of advice—do it while you can. In later years, such opportunities occur less frequently, but it always brings a smile to your face when you can reminisce about those times. Sometimes remembering your past exploits can bring on a rush of desire that leads to sudden sex—a quickie.

Here are some ideas about places to have sex other than the bed.

- **The Great Outdoors**—Although camping in the wilderness is definitely a fun change of sexual scenery, you can enjoy the outdoors in your own backyard too! Pitch a tent (pun intended) and share a sleeping bag.

- **The Couch**—Ladies, sit on the edge of the couch, so your hips are slightly off the edge, legs spread and feet on the floor. Have your guy kneel in front of you and enter you. You can move up and down, using your hands on his shoulders and feet against the floor. Alternatively, the man can sit on the couch and you can mount him as shown here.

- **The Weight Bench**—Put that weight bench in the basement to an added use. Guys, lay on your back, and let your woman straddle you and control the depth and pace.

- **The Dining Room**—Those armless chairs in your dining room are perfect for a little spontaneous sex. The man should sit on the chair, and like the cross-legged position, the woman sits on top of him, for a fun and different, but very intimate, location. Narrow, armless chairs in the living room work for this as well.

- **The Kitchen**—You may have heard, or read about having sex on the kitchen table—or counter top (it's more stable)—and this is a good way to raise the body, usually the female, to a level where the male has easier access to her vulva either for penetrative sex or cunilingus. The only problem here is that work surfaces and tables can be hard to lie on comfortably. Try a thin pillow or thick towel, to make the surface more comfortable.

- **The Couch 2**—The man sits on the couch or armchair, facing forward. The woman sits on his lap, allowing his penis to penetrate her from below, as seen in Figure 14. She leans forward slightly, his hands on her hips, as illustrated below. Her legs on the outside of his, gives the man more control of the movement. Her legs inside of his, gives a tighter feel and allows her to raise and lower herself on the man and gives her more control. Alternatively, the woman can sit facing the man, as shown in Figure 15, wrapping her legs around his torso. As you can see in the alternative positioning, this allows for great eye contact and kissing.

Figure 14: Couch 2 Position

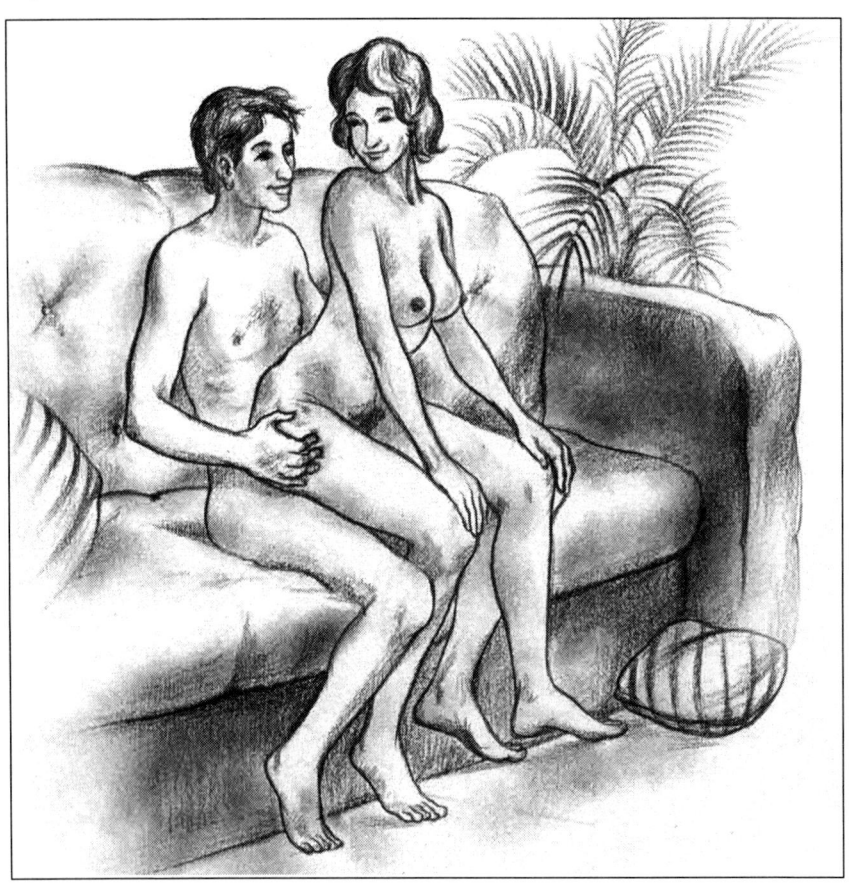

Figure 15: Couch 2 Position Alternative

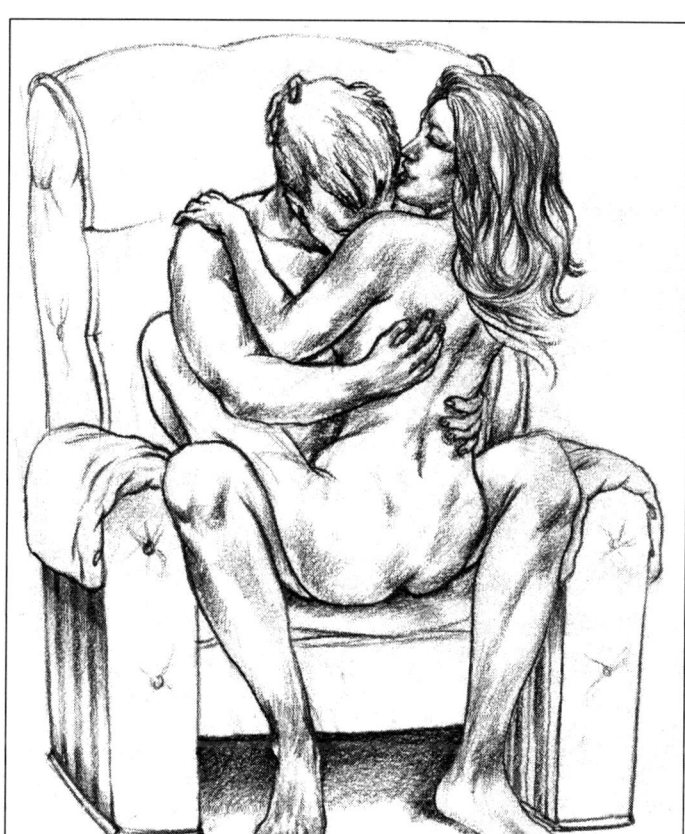

- **The Couch 3**—With the woman standing at the end of the couch or armchair, have her bend at the hips, over the arm of the couch. The man then enters her, while standing, from behind, as illustrated in Fig.16. If there is a significant height difference between the man or woman, one of you may have to stand on a book or firm pillow. If the man is taller, the alternative version of this position, as pictured below, with the woman kneeling on the couch or chair, can help offset the height difference.

Figure 16: Couch 3 Position

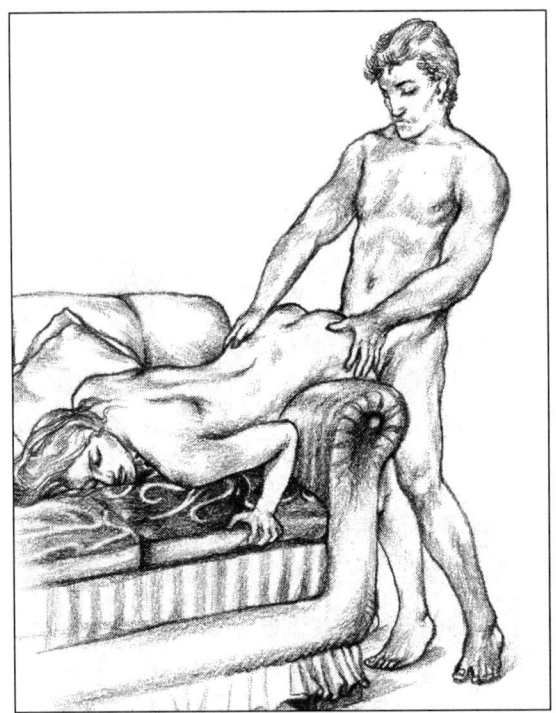

Figure 17: Couch 3 Position Alternative

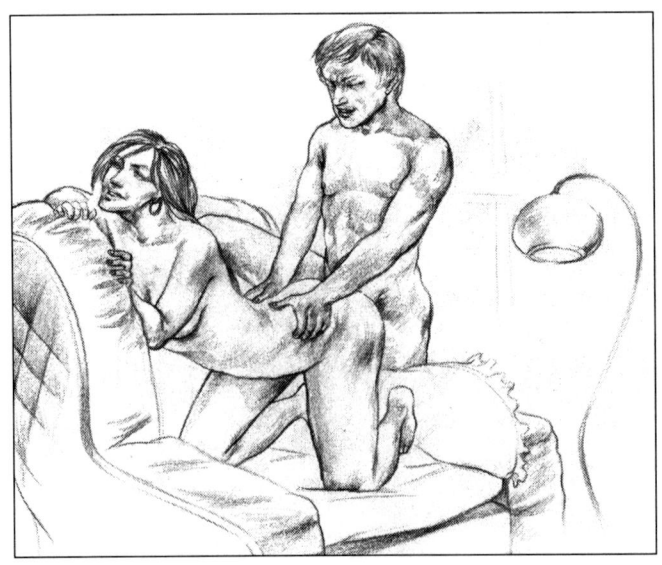

Regarding the Couch:

Although, you can use a sofa or armchair in many ways, I want to point out one of the advantages of using the arm at one end for sex, as illustrated. This is particularly beneficial, but not exclusively, for those guys who find thrusting positions not easy to maintain for as long as they would like. Men find it easier to maintain an erection, and reach orgasm, while standing up. This is a physiological phenomena and it becomes more apparent as you get older.

Making love can be pretty exhausting for either partner if prolonged in a position, or positions, needing physical exertion. Using the furniture can help to not only lessen the energy required but also help prolong the activity for the same reason. No matter where you have sex, there are three important things to remember:

Enjoy what you're doing.

Enjoy each other.

Never turn away from mutual desire.

—— 17 ——

Oral Sex

Clinton lied. A man might forget where he parks or where he lives, but he never forgets oral sex, no matter how bad it is.

~ Lenny Clarke

Kissing will often lead to kissing the most intimate parts. Tongues come into play. On the way down from her mouth, pause awhile over her breasts. Take little kisses toward a nipple. Gently caress the nipple with your tongue, and, if the reaction is inviting, cup the breast in your hand so that the nipple is prominent.

Girls, if you'd like to encourage him, use your own hand to cup your breast and offer it up to him. Likes and dislikes vary as much between females and males. Let him know if you like your nipples sucked, licked or pinched.

In my early sexual adventures, I had a liaison with a girl who wanted me to bite her nipples so hard, I was afraid I'd bite them off. Others can't stand biting. Each to their own. Just be sure to find out!

Next, trail your kisses from her navel to her thighs; leave the labia to the last. The teasing sensation will encourage her to guide you when she's ready for full-blown oral sex.

Giving Head

Going down on her or eating her out—these are familiar ways of describing cunnilingus. Guys, you should know that there are few women who do not like her man giving head. Think about it. How often would you refuse a woman who wanted to give you a blow-job?

There are some basic, and practical, aspects to consider, so I will give them a quick mention before we get down to it (pun intended).

- Hygiene and
- Position

Hygiene

I know it's obvious, but both men and women should try to anticipate the opportunity for oral sex and wash down there. As I've mentioned before, the sewer is only an inch away, and pubic hair is a perfect harbor for bacteria that develop weird odors.

Wash and rinse, then wash and rinse once more. Wash from the pubis right through and past the anus. Insert the tip of your index finger in the anus to ensure no deposits are left there. For maximum access, squat in the bathtub or shower while washing. Then dry with a clean fresh towel. Towels harbor bacteria, and it would be foolish to wash clean only to deposit new bacteria from the towel.

Those of us who use a bidet have reason to smile. We cannot understand why everybody doesn't have a bidet in the bathroom, as it helps in keeping this area clean. More information about bidets follows in a minute.

Position

Avoid the awkward body positions only a contortionist would be comfortable with. If you'd like, don't be afraid to whisper, "I'd love to go down on you." Immediately, this can signal both partners to rearrange their bodies to allow for this. There are a variety of oral sex positions you can try that don't require the limberness of a gymnast. Here are a few:

- **Woman on the Bed; Man on the Floor**—She lies across the bed, with her legs over the side. He kneels on the floor beside the bed, so she can raise her legs and rest them on his shoulders. He can use his hands to elevate her legs, with knees bent and parted, to provide access to the complete vulva area. His hands are also free to caress the underside of her thighs or use fingers to part her lips.

- **Both on the Bed**—He lies on the bed on his stomach, so his head can lie comfortably between her legs. If he cups her hips in his hands, his elbows taking his weight on the bed, he can adjust the position of his head and sense her reactions. If she wants to bend her knees and bring her thighs up, he can move his hands to the underside of her thighs, caress them or help spread them to maximize his access to the whole area. A pillow placed under her buttocks will raise her pubis and make the vulva even more inviting. It will also encourage her to thrust her pelvis forward and upwards towards his mouth when she finds his attentions stimulating.

- **Soixante-Neuf or 69**—The man lies in a position where the man's head is in line with her vulva and the woman's head is in line with his penis—we'll get to the blow-job in a minute. The most comfortable position for this will depend on the relative body sizes of the man and the woman. Most often the woman is smaller than the man, and for them it may be best for him on his back with her on top. She can move on to her knees to take her weight off his chest and open up her vulva at the same time. Try reversing this, with the woman underneath, but the guy should be sure to take his weight on his knees and elbows outside of her body. The only disadvantage of 69 is the man's mouth and tongue are primarily targeting only the clitoris. (See Figure 13: Sixty-Nine Position in Chapter 16.)

Bidets

As mentioned, having access to a bidet is an excellent way to stay as clean as possible, for oral sex. Chances are, if you've traveled through Europe, Latin America, the Middle East, East Asia, or China, you've encountered a bidet in the bathroom. A bidet is traditionally a basin, near the toilet, that's used to clean the genitals and anal area after using the toilet, or whenever a "freshening up" is needed. Using a bidet is easy!

- **First, straddle the bidet.** The big advantage of using a bidet is the position over the bidet ensures the entire area of your genitals and anus are exposed for washing. On most standalone bidets, you can either face the bidet's water controls or you can face away from them, as you would a toilet. Be sure that you know where the water will be coming from ahead of time, or you could end up with a surprise shower. If your bidet does have a spray nozzle set in the bowl (unlikely in the UK due to regulations), place your hand above it to subdue any jet of water and then either press or pull the diverter lever between or immediately behind the taps.

- **Second, clean the anal area and/or genitals.** Clean the desired area using your hands, as you would when taking a shower. This is another advantage with bidets. Both of your hands are free to do the washing/soaping. If you wish to use soap, use only those that are unscented since perfumed ones are not recommended for use on the genitals. Rinse yourself well and turn off the water.

- **Lastly, dry your skin.** Some bidets have a built-in air dryer that you can use. For others, simply pat dry with toilet paper. Many bidets have a towel on a ring positioned next to the bidet. This is for drying the genitals or the hands but sometimes it is used for mopping up any splashes around the rim after rinsing it.

Some additional benefits of using a bidet include:

1. People with limited mobility, such as the elderly, disabled, or ill can use a bidet to maintain cleanliness, when using a bathtub or shower is uncomfortable or dangerous.

2 They are especially helpful for people with hemorrhoids, since they reduce the amount of repetitive wiping that is needed.

3. The use of a bidet can help women when menstruating and prevent or minimize the occurrence of yeast infections or vaginitis.

4. You can use a bidet to quickly wash your feet. This is a standing joke among the British. The unspoken assumption is made that those who think a bidet is for washing your feet really need to be enlightened when it comes to all things sexual!

Countries especially known for having bidets, include: South Korea, Japan, Egypt, Greece, Italy, Spain, France, Portugal, Turkey, Argentina, Brazil, Uruguay, Venezuela, Lebanon, and India. There are many more countries where you will find them in increasing numbers, including the UK, and frequently installed in luxury hotels.

My grateful thanks for most of the above information to the contributors to

How To Use a Bidet, which can be found at: http://www.wikihow. com/Use-a-Bidet. There's even a short instructional video.

If, like most Americans, you don't have access to a bidet, the hand—held shower is a great alternative. Although you won't have use of both hands, a washcloth can help you ensure you get clean.

Oral Technique

Forget what you may have seen in porn; flicking the clitoris with your tongue is not a good idea—in the beginning.

Remember the wishbone analogy? With all those nerve endings down through the labia, on both sides of her vulva, you have a plethora of flesh to excite. With your mouth open (not too wide) plant your lips over her labia and gently rock your head from side to side. Her clitoris should be just above your upper lip. She will want you to move up to her clitoris and may even grab your head to guide you, but resist teasingly for a few moments while you pass your extended tongue in a gentle sweeping motion, from the lower end of her vulva up as far as the clitoris. Make your tongue as flat as you can against her moist opening with this motion and resist penetrating her vagina.

Repeat this move very slowly, but concentrate on one side nibbling the labia as you go. When you nibble cup your upper teeth inside your upper lip or lower with lower lip, whichever you find easiest—no biting with teeth here, please. Return your extended tongue to the lower end and do the same motion to the other side. By now, you should be noticing some change in her labia. They will swell with blood as she is stimulated.

Next, start from the lower end again and move up just a little and pause while you tickle the entrance to her vagina with the tip of your tongue. If you happen to be blessed with a very long tongue, let it enter. Dextrous use of your fingers may gently part her lips at this point, so that the surrounding area to her vagina is exposed. Massage this area with your tongue.

Now move up as before and lay your tongue flat against her clitoris. Gently rock your head from side to side. She will take this for as long as you like. Don't try to raise her hood with the tip of your tongue until she is absolutely ready for it. She will give you all kinds of indication when she wants change.

Stay aware of her breathing and body movements. If she starts thrusting her hips into your face, you will know you're on the right path. Whenever the indications are right, don't change what you're doing. Don't change speed, just keep the pressure and pace, and she will have a clitoral climax.

This is not an exact science. We're all different, and we all have different desires at different times. There are many aspects to giving good head, not least how well you know your partner and how well you communicate with each other. There will be times when the woman will be content to lie there and enjoy the experience without climaxing. There will be times when she will arrive at the point of orgasm within a few minutes. There will also be times when she will want you to "take her completely," with penetrative sex using your penis.

If you're inexperienced at oral sex, or have tried it and didn't enjoy it, my message is—Persevere!

Good oral sex is as good as it gets. If at first you find the different textures, smells, fluids, and warmth of a vagina challenging, try dip-and—dive. Dive down there, dip briefly with your tongue, and retreat. However, be sure to repeat and stay down there a little longer each time. You will soon start to enjoy it—I promise! Ask her to help you to give her what she likes. The rewards are amazing.

Blow Jobs

The more formal term for blow jobs is fellatio. In general, the woman gives head to the man by taking his penis in her mouth and brings him to orgasm by using her lips, tongue, mouth, and movement. No blowing involved but maybe a little sucking and nibbling.

Let's ask Batwoman what she thinks about oral sex.

> *One of the reasons that I LOVE oral sex is my mouth is much more sensitive than my vagina, and I can feel a lot*

more when a man cums in my mouth. Orally, I can get it all—the feeling of his cock pulsing and pumping, the hot cum fountaining out and filling my mouth and throat, and the taste and heat of it. Many more sensations than I get vaginally. I really like that!

When I was younger, I thought that for oral to be good for the man, the woman needed to move her mouth up and down his shaft constantly. Now, I know better. There are lots of other things that can be added into the mix, especially right at the end. Things I like to do include:

1. Moving my mouth up and down over his whole shaft.

2. Staying still while he thrusts into my mouth (I often like to wrap my hand around the base of his cock, so I can control the depth of his thrusts).

3. Holding him still in my mouth while I swirl my tongue around his glans and tease his frenulum with my tongue.

4. Having him stroke his shaft (preferably well lubed) with his hand, while I suck and tease his glans.

5. Stroking his shaft with my hand, while I suck and tease his glans.

I enjoy the last two particularly, because I can control his depth in my mouth and throat and feel the excitement build, as he gets closer to cumming. It is truly remarkable how the emotional quotient can build there at the end, and that feels lovely in my mouth!

When he finally starts to tip over the point of no return, he and/or I can keep stroking, while I hold the head of his cock in my mouth as he cums. That way the stimulation doesn't stop for him, but at the same time I get to feel and experience everything his cock is doing while he cums. This is a major thrill for me.

Advice from Abby of *I Teach Blow Jobs*

Abby runs a blog she calls, *I Teach Blow Jobs.* In the Summer of 2010, she wrote this piece of advice, "One thing that I constantly hear from detractors of blow jobs is that they are degrading toward women.

Obviously these people don't understand how oral sex works."

Remember, every guy is different. I can't say this enough.

Just because your ex loved your blow jobs, it doesn't mean every guy will. Some guys love things that other guys hate. They have different amounts of sensitivity in different areas. They like different techniques, different speed and pressures, and even this can even be true of a single guy over time. The advice I give should always be treated as if it carries the disclaimer:

Will work for most guys, most of the time.

This is why it's important to have wide-ranging experiences and learn as much as you can. Even if you only plan on being with one guy forever, he can change, and he might like things neither of you have ever even considered.

One thing is fairly universal—guys like blow jobs. Even a bad blow job is better than nothing at all, and guys are not going to tell you if it was bad. The reason is simple—if they do, there's a good chance it won't happen again.

Don't let the guys telling you how great you are go to your head (no pun intended). Ninety-nine percent of the time a guy will tell you it was great or the best they've had. Even when they promise they're being "completely honest," or it's a close friend or long-time partner, guys will often exaggerate your skill level to avoid hurting your feelings. It's a sad fact that guys themselves are the main reason most women don't get any better at giving head.

Before you decide to believe what you've been told about your blow job prowess, think about it seriously and consider this—my personal estimates are that the average woman barely begins to develop her own technique until she's given between 50 and 100 blow jobs. She doesn't really start getting good until she's done at least 200. Lastly, she doesn't hit the level of amazing any guy will tell her she is, until around blow job number 1,000.

At first, that sounds like a lot. However, if you're seeing a guy and blowing him three times a week, which isn't really that much, that's over 150 blow jobs per year. If you keep that up from age 20, you'll hit 1000 by your late-20s.

Wetter is Better

Funny thing about stimulating a guy—friction is what creates the pleasure, but by lubricating and therefore reducing friction, the pleasure is increased. I have no idea what the scientific basis is for this, but it works.

Saliva is generally a good thing. It's a plentiful, natural lubricant that combines with pre-seminal fluid in a ridiculously, efficient way to create a natural super-lubricant that is almost always enough for the simplest blow job. However, if you want to have breast sex or do a lot with your hands (in short, if you want to give the best blow jobs possible) you should invest in a commercial lubricant. Get something flavored and make sure it tastes OK to you, before you go lathering him up.

Don't Twiddle Your Thumbs

How much do you use your hands in day-to-day life? Chances are it's a lot. Without our physiological dexterity and patented opposable thumbs, we humans would still be wandering around in swamps wondering how to grab that stick over there.

Unless you need to use a hand to keep balance or maintain comfort, you should be using both hands at all times in some way. You don't have to be using them to give an actual hand-job. You can rub other erogenous zones, cup the testes, trail your fingers lightly across his abdomen or inside of his thighs, or do anything your hands can usefully do. It can actually take a bit of practice to get all of your mouth and hand movements properly in rhythm with one another, but it's worth getting right. Your hands are to a blow job what cranberry sauce is to roast turkey. It's not strictly necessary, but it makes it so much better.

Use All of Your Mouth

Too many women have the attitude just putting a penis in their mouth is enough. They think the mouth is a replacement for the vagina. As long as things go in and out in succession, everything is fine. The fact is, your mouth has a lot more hardware in it.

Saying your mouth is like your vagina is the same as saying your computer is like your calculator. Your mouth has a tongue, teeth and lips, all of which are unique to that part of your body. Your tongue feels different than the roof of your mouth, and both are different again to your inner cheeks. Each surface feels different to the guy, and each has a role it can play during the blow job.

The Figure Eight

A simple technique that shows off the variety of the mouth is the Figure Eight. Take the penis part or all of the way into your mouth and create a seal with your lips. You don't want to make the seal too strong. Keep some movement. Now, trace a sideways figure eight (or infinity sign) in the air with your nose, while you allow the penis to slide around the inside of your mouth. Pay attention to his reactions, and don't be afraid to ask him what he thought afterward.

We all know teeth are usually bad during a blow job. However, some light nibbling can be good. Some guys even like you to apply a bit of pressure, especially with the flatter molars at the back of the mouth. Teeth are like terrorism; be aware but not alarmed.

Get Over It

You are not the first person to ever give head, and it's not some clandestine act that only happens in secret caverns during a full moon. A huge part of oral sex is psychological. Once you can get over the societal taboos and indoctrination associated with it, you will be a much better and happier fellatrix.

Being honest and open about it is one of the first steps along that path. Discuss it with a friend or a professional. Most importantly, don't be afraid to admit you do it. After all, nearly everyone does.

Enjoy It

The most important rule to great blow jobs is to enjoy doing it! The more you like it, the better you'll be at it.

Journaling

Buy a blow job journal. Use it to keep a record of your experiences—where, when, and who. Did you try anything new? What did or didn't work? Is there anything you feel you can take away from the experience to make yourself a better fellatrix? The bottom line—you can only be as good as you work to be.

The Basics

Have you ever noticed the attitudes men have towards their genitalia? To most, it is the symbol of masculinity, sometimes even a representation of their own self. I know a lot of guys who call their penis

Little (insert guy's name here). In one case, a guy we'll call Jim referred quite accurately to his ten-inch anaconda as 'Big Jim.' He was only a bit over five feet tall.

The genital area, the testes especially, is very sensitive. If you've seen a guy get hit in the balls, you know exactly what I'm talking about. The penis is also essential for proper urination, reproduction, sexual satisfaction, and writing one's name in the snow. The point I'm making here is a guy's cock is very important to him.

Now, take a look at your mouth. See all those teeth? They were designed to destroy things that go in your mouth. You have incisors for sharp cutting, canines for grip, and molars for crushing and pulverizing. You have a jaw, a surprisingly strong mass of muscle and bone, to power it all. In short, your mouth is always going to win a fight with any cock that might come its way. Add your hands into the equation and you are very much in charge.

Psychology and Body Language

Take the most iconic position for oral sex—the guy is standing, and the girl is on her knees. Kneeling is a submissive position. It implies obedience, even reverence. The guy is standing over her, implying he is her superior—the object of reverence.

There is no way around this, but you can skew it slightly. Worship the cock, not the man. The act of oral sex is on one level a demonstration of adoration for the penis. It's sometimes best to forget the guy, and just concentrate on his cock.

The Guy's Perspective

Whatever is going on, if a man can see it, it will always speed up and heighten his excitement. For this reason, there is a good position for the woman that not only allows the man to see what she's doing but also is key in communication between them. It also definitely puts the woman in charge of the event. This position is where the guy lies on his back across the bed, with his feet on the floor and knees wide apart. His girl kneels on the floor, between his knees and faces him.

From this position, she can apply her mouth and tongue wherever the feeling takes her. In addition, there are three other advantages:

- She can maintain eye contact with him. Don't worry if he closes his eyes now and then. This will only be a result of the ecstasy he feels.

- The next advantage requires a little reminder of his physiology. If left alone lying on his back, his fully erect penis will always lie flat against his belly. This is where the penile ligaments take it. Take his penis in your hand and bring it upright, so it's in a better position for you to place in your mouth. You will feel this action going against the pull of those ligaments. This exerts a strong, additional feeling of excitement for a man.

- In this position, holding his penis upright, you are directly facing the most sensitive part of his penis: the frenulum. You can drive him mad with your tongue, thumb, nipple, breasts, or whatever you want at this angle.

Tasty Semen

Seminal fluid has its own unique texture and flavor. The texture ranges, as described by Dr Christian Jessen in Chapter 8: The Chemistry of Love & Lust, from gloopy to watery, and the color also varies from milky white to a pale gray. Taking these varying textures in the mouth can be challenging for some—there's nothing quite like the texture of seminal fluid!

Apart from texture, taste is what can make it attractive or loathsome. The better the taste, the easier it is for your partner to accept the unique texture. I think it is true to say it is an acquired taste—some girls just love it; others find it repulsive. Here's where guys can help make the act of taking semen in their mouth more acceptable to your lover—and therefore offer this very special act to you more readily, and maybe more frequently!

"You are what you eat." Where have I heard that before? This is true for semen. What you eat affects the taste of your semen. In fact, other things you take into your body also affect semen flavor. Not exactly edible, but just as influential, is tobacco smoke. If your lover is a smoker, you already know how bitter his semen tastes.

If your lover has a sweet tooth and eats lots of fresh sweet fruit, like strawberries, his semen will take on a hint of fruity flavor. You can guess what garlic and onions do! Try and keep to a healthy diet with plenty of fresh fruit, a wide variety of vegetables—avoiding spicy ones, as well as bitter nuts—and avoid alcoholic drinks but stick to fresh still water, and you (or rather, she) will notice the changes in taste over the weeks.

Thankfully, some foods described as aphrodisiacs contain flavonoids, which are good for you and can actually influence the taste of your semen. Check out the list of flavonoids in the Aphrodisiacs section of Chapter 8: The Chemistry of Love and Lust.

More Advice from Abby

Let's get back to Abby. Here's her specific advice.

Taking it Like a Woman

You've done all the hard work. Whether it's taken you a few minutes or a couple of hours, you've worked his cock right up to the brink and now he's about to cum. If you're doing it right, you're going to be in this situation a lot. Beyond the academic 'spit versus swallow' argument, you probably haven't given it much thought.

Getting Over the Edge

A point is eventually reached during a blow job where orgasm becomes inevitable. His breathing becomes short and the head inflates—you know the drill. There are a few schools of thought regarding stimulation in and around the moment of eruption. Some guys have different preferences, but I recommend keeping up whatever you're doing as the guy cums. After the first couple of spurts, slow it down and gradually stop. If the guy wants more or less stimulation, you can usually tell from his reactions.

A Comment from an Abby Reader

I'm going to leave the last word to a man who responded to Abby's post with the following comment.

> *I enjoy a lady who wants me to cum in her mouth, so she can share some of it with me in a kiss, and we can both swallow it at the same time. Either that, or have me cum on her breasts so we can feed it to each other from our fingers after she milks my cock dry with her lips.*

The Perfect Finish

Time taken to arrive at the perfect finish can be anywhere from two to 20 minutes. My view of an ideal blow job time for a lucky man is approximately nine to ten minutes. Much longer and the poor girl will not only have an aching face but also sore lips and mouth. If it is going to take longer, don't be surprised if she moves from using her mouth to just using her hands.

The situation, time and place will all affect the amount of time taken. The excitement and danger of doing it in a public place (not that I'm recommending this), for instance, can raise the level of excitement to fever pitch and, especially for a young man, can cause a sudden rush. Also, for the young man, the circumstances and only a little physical contact can do the job.

As we get a little older and more in control, we can deliberately bring on the orgasm when we feel the time is right. The woman can sense this moment. She feels his body tense, his breathing become shallow and the final extra hardening of his penis in her mouth immediately preceding his ejaculation.

By the time we reach our 60's, 70's and beyond, comfort is the key. The man being fellated will probably choose a comfortable chair, if not the bed. His partner kneels on the floor and faces him between his legs. This way, she can lean on his thighs. He can use his hands to caress her neck and shoulders, and she can indicate when it's time to finish with her eyes. Incidentally, if her breasts are just touching his knees, this can be a very erotic feeling for both partners.

This is the time when most men fantasize. They concentrate on something in their minds they find erotic, simply to bring on the ejaculation. Now, I want to stress to the female reader that this does not mean he finds you anything less than his perfect partner. It is simply a mechanism men use to reach the point of no return.

Every man has a different fantasy. It can vary from a whole range of visions and activities, and that's why it's best described as fantasy. In other words, it is never real. Be reassured, and don't worry if he prefers not to talk about them. Although it can be a lot of fun to share fantasies with each other!

When he's about to ejaculate, even when you're expecting it, the actual first spurt always seems to come as a surprise to the woman. A little understanding of seminal fluid can be helpful. Opinions differ among women on the topic.

Some find it erotic and just love it. Others find it objectionable and will always ensure it lands nowhere near their face. My own view is it is the consistency of ejaculate that makes it so different to anything else we might have enter our mouths.

There is no doubt, for the man, tensing up and feeling the rush through several spasms—usually four to six but in rare cases as many as ten or 11—of his semen going into her mouth is the most amazing feeling. Because he will naturally want to thrust upwards at the point of no return, and the woman doesn't wish to have his penis disappear down her throat, she should grasp his penis around the base of his shaft, so she remains in control of his thrust.

Keeping her lips around his glans and tip of her tongue sliding against the frenulum, she can maintain a gentle in and out motion while he cums. Her lips needn't go any further down than just past his glans. She will feel each spurt on her tongue. Don't worry about it filling your mouth; the actual total volume is never going to be more than a teaspoon. Keep the movement going until well past his last spasm. This is a short period of awesome, whole body thrill of pleasure for the man.

Alternatively, she can hold her lips and mouth still over his penis and use her free hand to stroke the penis to orgasm. The woman will know when to stop, because she will feel his penis losing its hardness.

Following is an excellent alternative If you feel like you can't take your man's penis in your mouth without gagging.

- First, take it easy and play with your lips around his glans to begin with.

- Then experiment with allowing a little more to enter your mouth and withdraw.

- Do this a few times; then go a little deeper, but stop before you feel the gagging reflex.

- Use your tongue and nibble gently down the length of his shaft and back to the glans in your mouth once more.

- Pinching the loose skin of his scrotum and pulling down adds to his pleasure.

For the man lucky enough to enjoy a blow job from a partner who can take the entire length of his penis in her mouth, the sensation for him is as close as he will ever get to heaven. However, the loving partner will always be thinking of what both can enjoy with this exercise. The man who forces his penis down her throat and holds her head, in order to do so, is in no way a lover. Indeed, I would describe this as rape.

In the end, the woman has a spoonful of cum in her mouth. What should she do with it?

Once more, we're all different. I know of one woman who doesn't swallow because it gives her indigestion. As another pointed out to me, "Taking it in my mouth and swallowing are two totally different experiences." There are many things you can do with a mouthful of cum, but the reasonable and loving partner won't mind at all if his girl simply wipes it away on a tissue.

Time for Sleep

It is at this point the man's cerebral cortex shuts down. When he's finished the *cingulate cortex* and *amygdale* tell the rest of the brain to deactivate from sexual desire. This is accompanied by a surge of chemicals, such as oxytocin and serotonin, which can have a powerful sleep-inducing effect.

According to Neuroscientist, Serge Stoleru, whose research is published in the journal *Neuroscience and Biobehavioral Reviews,*

> *Our experiments give us the first hints as to what happens in the brain during orgasm. After men have an orgasm they usually experience a refractory period when they cannot get aroused. For women it seems to be different. They don't seem to have such a strong refractory period and may be asking for more when their partners just want a rest.*[106]

One of the chemicals released is prolactin, which is linked to the feeling of sexual satisfaction. Earlier research has found men who are deficient in prolactin are less tired after orgasm.[107]

Dr. Stoleru added, "The human brain is involved in all the successive steps of sexual behavior."[108] It may be a relief for some women to know there is a biological explanation for the roll-over-and-sleep effect.

—— 18 ——

Anal Sex

A man must have confidence in himself and his cock, to fuck a woman in the ass. If he does not have this control, his cock will direct the action; he will move too quickly, hurt the once-willing woman, and rarely, rightly, will he be given a second chance.

~ Toni Bentley

It's All About Trust

Before we even think about anything involving our anus, it is understood, for cultural or religious reasons, many of you will want to skip this section. I also recognize, for many, this will be the first time you have ventured in this direction. It may be just out of curiosity, or it may be because you've always wanted to try it, or your partner may be interested in anal sex but not you.

There are many questions, and I will try to cover most. However, please don't consider what follows to be comprehensive or necessarily right for you. Remember, we're all different!

This chapter should be taken as a guide and introduction to the basic essentials of anal sex, so you can avoid the many pitfalls and misconceptions that result from total ignorance and the taboos instilled by centuries of unenlightened social pressures. If you follow the comments made by those quoted here with experience in anal sex, and communicate your deepest thoughts and desires to the one you love—and this DEFINITELY has to be two-way communication—over time, you should discover the best moves to suit you both. This can make anal sex as joyous as any other sexual activity you choose.

It Should Never Hurt

If anything about anal sex hurts, you're not doing it right!

Even and ESPECIALLY the first time. It should NOT hurt. The anus and its sphincter, which holds it tight shut, are packed with nerve endings that easily detect pain, just as these nerves also easily convey pleasure when treated right. Inside the rectum is a thin-walled tube that is easily damaged. For this reason, anything we do down there has to be delicately performed.

Here are a few things you should note:

- **ALWAYS** go about anal sex slowly. Always.

- **ALWAYS** lubricate and use plenty of it. Unlike the vagina, the rear end is not self-lubricating. Choose a water soluble lube—baby oil may be fine for other areas but always use a water-based lube for anal. If in doubt, talk to your pharmacist. Baby oil degrades condoms but water-based lubes don't, and your rectum prefers water to oil anytime.

- **MANICURED** hands and nails are essential. Torn anal tissue is not only painful, it is dangerous. It is the most vulnerable area to infection. Don't be shy to use a surgical glove or a condom to cover your finger or fingers, if it makes you or your partner safer.

- **TALK** to each other constantly and openly. Communication and absolute trust are essential.

- **NEVER** surprise her; she must always be prepared for what you are about to do.

- **NEVER** use a desensitizing cream, on your penis or your/her anus. Don't use a condom treated with a desensitizer either. You both want to feel and enjoy the sensations.

- **NEVER** take your penis out of her anus and insert it into her vagina; this is just asking for serious bacterial infection. The same goes for sucking a penis that has just been in the ass—never, ever do it.

Here's some commonsense evidence, as reported by Ky Henderson, on YourTango.com:

> *Experts estimate one in four straight couples have had anal sex, arguably making it the most popular of sexual taboos. However, while many people are at the very least curious enough to try it, few go about it the right way. The result? They have a negative experience and never do it again.*[109]

> *In order to enjoy anal sex, couples need to have some idea of what they're doing, and must communicate with each other. Of course, talking frankly about a ding-dong in a yoo-hoo can be tough. "Our asses carry with them so much cultural baggage," says Tristan Taormino, author of The Ultimate Guide to Anal Sex For Women. "Most of us are taught at a young age that our butts are dirty, that they shouldn't be shared with others, that they are not a source of pleasure—all of which aren't true."*[110]

> *Despite that (or perhaps because of it), the idea of anal sex is often a turn-on. Men like the promise of tightness and friction, and both partners can appreciate the allure of unique physical sensations coupled with domination/ submission. Think those qualities make it deviant?*[111]

Maybe so, but they also make it intensely intimate. As porn star Jenna Jameson wrote of anal sex in her 2004 autobiography, "I've only given that up to three men, all of whom I really loved. Doing it on camera would be compromising myself."[112]

Here's more information, as reported on the NetDoctor website:

The Taboo of Anal Sex

Anal sex is one of the most taboo forms of sexual intercourse. Anal sex goes hand-in-hand, for many, with feelings of guilt, moral indignation and anxiety. However, as noted above, it's one of the most commonly practiced sexual taboos. Although some may find the idea of this act repugnant, others find it exciting and a normal part of their sex life.

Whether we're comfortable with the idea of anal sex or not, the anus is naturally equipped with erotic nerve endings, in both women and men. For this reason, it's not a surprise that so many couples (both heterosexual and homosexual) get pleasure from anal stimulation, despite the taboo.

Who Does It?

The most common societal misconception about anal sex is that it is practiced mostly by gay men. Not so! In fact, not only do many heterosexual couples enjoy anal sex, but it's been reported that nearly 1/3 of gay couples do NOT use anal sex in their sex lives, and 10 percent of heterosexual couples practice anal sex regularly in their lovemaking. When comparing actual numbers of people having anal sex, more heterosexual couples have anal sex than homosexual couples, since there are more heterosexual couples in general.[113]

Batwoman's contribution during a PEGym.com forum discussion on anal sex noted:

I happen to quite enjoy anal sex . . . . but it took a lot of years for me to discover that, and a partner who was very patient and concerned that I enjoy ALL parts of what we were doing.

First off, communication is key. You both have to get over any embarrassment about it, and talk about what you are doing. For me, having him invite me to explore him anally as well was a good introduction. Lots of lube (or soap in the shower) and fingertip play can go a long way toward making you both comfortable. Be sure to have a sense of humor about it—don't get all serious or demanding, just introduce anal play as something fun to experiment with each others bodies.

Pain Free

Lube, lube, lube. This is what makes anal play and anal sex fun. Nobody likes something large and unlubricated inserted anally—it hurts.

GOOD ANAL SEX IS PAIN-FREE.

I cannot emphasize this enough.

If it hurts at all, she is not ready enough or not lubed enough. This goes for whether or not you are inserting your finger or your cock. It takes time and lube and a lot of massaging to get the anus to relax enough for penetration (of any kind) to feel good.

Never Rush

Never, ever rush anything. Make sure she knows if she wants you to stop or back off, you will. If you try some sort of "oops" routine, she will know that you cannot be trusted, and this will damage both your relationship and any chance you might have had to get her to like anal sex.

If she seems to enjoy having you massage her anus and insert a fingertip during sex, I expect that she would enjoy more. But take it slowly. It may take quite a number of exploratory sessions before she is ready to even think about letting you try to insert your cock. The best thing that you can do is work on getting her to like your finger. Explore lubes, and when she is receptive slowly insert a bit more of your finger, being sure to massage around in a circle as you press inward. GO SLOWLY.

Mutual Pleasure

When I was learning about my ass, my guy waited until I was essentially begging for him to try sliding his cock inside. He let me take the lead and let me decide what position I was most comfortable in. He let me decide when we would try more than just finger play.

That meant a lot to me. It made it something that we did together for mutual pleasure, not something that he did to me. It also ensured that I was really truly ready the first time we tried actual anal sex.

Advanced Sex

I guess I really don't see anal play and anal sex as a "mainstream fetish" at all—just an extension of intimacy and sexuality into a slightly new anatomical area. In retrospect, it seems really weird to me that I was always free to touch any part of my lover's body EXCEPT this small region, which was somehow off-limits . . . . and vice versa.

What a wonderful surprise to discover that it feels good to touch, and be touched, there! As for penetration, that takes time, preparation and, above all else, trust. Trust is key.

Anal sex is definitely advanced sex—not for beginners or for couples who are even a little unsure of their sexuality, initimacy or trust levels. It also requires a substantial time commitment (you cannot have quickie anal sex). But you can have anal play anytime.

Now that I have discovered anal play, it is one of my favorite things. By "anal play" I mean touching and caressing the anus, with gentle insertion of a fingertip or finger. We do this all the time as part of regular sex—he does it with me and I with him. He loves it when I suck his cock while playing with his ass; I love it when he massages me while stroking me or when we are having sex doggie style (thus exposing my anus for gentle stimulation by his fingers during vaginal sex). We also enjoy playing with each other in the shower, when there is lots of slippery skin and soap suds to make it all feel great.

I also enjoy full-blown anal sex—his hard cock in my ass. Not all the time, but sometimes it is exactly what I want. Yes, I ask for it. Why not? I see no benefits of being shy in the bedroom.

From the uninitiated female perspective, anal sex can definitely seem like something that is only for the guy—he wants it, he pressures you for it and, if you give in, the best you can hope for is that it won't hurt and won't be messy. The reality can be far different and a source of great pleasure for women too, but it takes the right partner and the right time to make it so.

Deeply Erotic

Have I ever had an orgasm from anal sex? No, not from that alone, but I have had great orgasms during anal sex from using a vibrator on my clit.

Does anal feel different from vaginal sex? You bet! It is deeply erotic in a different way; it's hard to describe. I enjoy the fullness and the stretching when he is deep inside me. It is very, very intimate and very, very erotic. It took a lot of years for us to discover it, but I think my partner would also agree that it is wonderful addition to our sexuality and sex lives.

Personally I suspect that almost anyone would enjoy anal play, were they not hung up on misconceptions about it.

As you read this, you might be wondering how it is women claim to enjoy anal sex, yet, unlike the vagina, there are no erogenous zones within to be stimulated.

Having read so far, you can see it isn't just anal penetration that provides pleasure, it is invariably a combination of stimulating other areas at the same time. It doesn't have to be with a vibrator. Your partner has fingers, and you have fingers—use them!

However, I do have some more good news. The wall of the rectum is very thin and right next to the vagina. This means stimulation of the vaginal erogenous zones can be achieved via the rectum. It's just a question of depth—and this is where some experimentation is necessary in order to achieve the right positions for you and your partner.

The A-Spot Revisited

We have previously talked about the A-spot and how deep it is when approached by a finger in the vagina. In fact, many folk discover they can't reach it, so don't be surprised if this happens to you. However, because of the proximity of the vaginal wall to the rectum, and the angle at which it sits, it is possible to stimulate the A-spot via the anus with the added advantage of not hitting the cervix, which many women find painful.

With this in mind, we now have the prospect of deep vaginal orgasm, by stimulating the A-spot or alternatively, and not so deep, G-spot stimulation. This is in addition to clitoral orgasm brought on by using his or her fingers, while the man's penis does little more than rest deep inside her. This gives her that 'full' feeling and gently stimulates her A-spot with the head of his penis. We'll discuss this in greater depth later.

Prepping for Anal Sex

In the heat of passion, it is easy to forget simple preparations to avoid awkward or embarrassing situations following your love-making. By the time you have both lost all inhibitions, realize there is the possibility of just a little 'poo' appearing. For this reason, it's a good idea to lay a towel over the bed before you begin.

An old, large bath towel is best. It's simple to roll up and put in the washing machine afterward. A towel can even be used by the lady as a signal she's really up for it, by laying it out across the bed before he enters the bedroom!

Such a device can be given a nickname—you choose one—so you can refer to it in public without anyone else knowing what you're talking about (see the Communication chapter). In a restaurant, over a romantic dinner, you might say to your partner: "Since we're not working tomorrow, we should go for a jog before breakfast." In this instance, the 'jog' would be your favorite towel!

Here's an extract from a blog discussion on ways to prep your butt for anal sex:

From blog respondent, Skeptical:

> *Although my man doesn't know how I "prepare" for his occasional butt dips, I realize now my method works best for me. I never knew there were ways to achieve the "clean" butt. Common sense just told me I would always need a clean butt before penetration! I thought my method of cleaning inside my butt in the shower was weird and should never be said out loud! But damn!! I'm not strange!*
>
> *Some people go through great lengths, apparently. I decided to search the net to see if there was a real way to prepare myself, but apparently there are many methods of "rocket science" and all of them don't sound so clean! I'm relieved that I'm not weird.*
>
> *I think everyone needs to find a way that suits them. The last thing I want to do is poop on my man or have a smell going on. He'd love me anyway, but I'd rather NOT. The shower, soap and finger work well for me. The only thing that upsets me is I must be prepared for this. I can't have spontaneous anal sex which bums me out. Oh well.*

The debate continued. Here's what Bottomsup had to say:

> *It pays to know a little about our anatomy. Men and women are the same in respect to their bottoms.*
>
> *The anal canal is about three inches long and contains no poop. Next comes the rectum, which is between six and eight inches long and is normally empty until it fills up with poop from the colon. When this happens, a feeling of fullness results and an urge to go to the toilet results, in order to empty it again. If the rectum is empty, there is no danger of strong pooy smells or even smells at all.*
>
> *Some people feel they need the toilet when the rectum begins to fill, but others less fortunate, or who simply put the*

matter off, will have a rectum that is quite full without really noticing it. A full rectum will make anal sex very messy and smelly. The answer is to see to it that the rectum is empty.

The rectum is normally emptied by a bowel movement or should be washed out with water in the form of a small enema of no more than half a pint or so, held for several minutes. The reason for this? If a large enema is taken, water will travel up the colon washing down brown water and smelly poop at intervals for up to an hour afterward. Brown water being forced out during anal sex is not much fun for either party.

Probably, the best overall method is to train the bowel to have a movement every day soon after breakfast and maybe again in the early evening. They say the bowel has a subsidiary "brain" of its own, and it will respond to training if a regular diet of decent food is eaten and plenty of water is drank, up to six or seven glasses a day.

Some people are very regular, and these may be the ones that have no trouble with anal, because they are usually "empty." Constipation is the biggest culprit for pooy sex, as the rectum is often full of hard matter which sticks when anal sex is practiced.

Anyone can check if the rectum is full or not by inserting a rectal thermometer or similar, into the rectum to about its full length and checking if the tip is pooy when withdrawn. If it is, the rectum is full. If the rectum is empty, the thermometer will be clean along its entire length.

In conclusion, I would also suggest that a condom be used at all times. I would also suggest that however smelly the anal intercourse is, the man should never show his disgust at the woman. After all, she is allowing an unnatural act, however pleasant, to be enacted on her body, and it seems unkind to me for the man to show any displeasure if there is a smell.

Just be glad of the pleasure and help in improving things in the future.

Another Practical Note

People often advise, like Bottomsup just did, to drink a certain number of glasses of water each day. However, they never say what size the glass should be. General medical practitioners suggest two liters of water every day, but go on to remind us that other drinks, like tea, coffee, lemonade, and even beer count toward the total. Some drinks, like those containing alcohol or caffeine, have a diuretic effect, so they can count against the total.

If you have a sensible, balanced diet, you will also be getting some fluid from the fresh fruit and green vegetables you eat. For this reason, walking around with a bottle of water in your hand all day really isn't necessary, unless you live in a dessert area! Incidentally, another reason to eat your greens—the folic acid in leafy vegetables, especially kale and spinach, increases histamine production in women, boosting their ability to orgasm.

I agree with Bottomsup about using a condom for anal sex. It substantially reduces the chance of infection and is easy to take off the penis immediately following withdrawal for discrete disposal. You might also consider using condoms especially designed for anal sex. They're a little tougher than regular condoms and reduce the risk of a condom split.

Regular Routine

In order to be completely confident you're not going to expel anything unpleasant in the thrill of orgasm, it's best to empty both your bowel and your bladder before you begin. If you defecate and urinate every morning, followed by washing your 'undercarriage,' as my flying friends refer to it, you can get into the habit of easing and cleaning your anus with your fingers. Here are some easy-to-follow steps:

- Get into the best position to thoroughly wash, from front to back, and all the way up to where your butt-crack begins

- Rinse with running water, using a hand-held shower head or using hands and running tap.

- Go back to the anus and insert the tip of a soapy finger.

- Do this three or four times.

- Your anus will start to relax, so you can insert a finger up to the first joint.

- Pull out and repeat.

- Rinse well again using the same finger technique.

- As the soap leaves your finger, you will notice that it is no longer as easy to penetrate, which is a reminder of the importance to lube when you are having anal play or penetration.

Once you get into the habit of making this an everyday ritual, you can soon follow one finger with two and turn them slightly, which will leave your anus squeaky clean. Plus, it only takes a couple of minutes.

Irrigation

You will read about people giving themselves an enema and even 'irrigating' their colon. If you're going to have an enema, the best place to be is in a hospital.

There are a number of ways you can self-administer an enema, as you will see from numerous blogging comments made about it, but you need to know just half-a-pint of warm water is sufficient to clean out your rectum. Also, an enema is only necessary as a last resort, if you are genuinely uncertain about your own bowel movements, and you don't want to risk the slightest show of poo on the end of his condom-covered penis when he takes it out. There is a degree of trial and error here.

Don't force the water in. When medically applied, medical professionals simply insert a flexible tube into the anus and let gravity take the water in. There are some enema bags with a rubber squeeze-ball to speed things up a little, and it's possible to use the large-diameter injector—style tubes designed to feed animals or babies who are unable to suck for themselves. However, you don't want to force the water in too fast. It will readily mix with whatever excrement is present, while you squeeze your ass tight and hold for a few minutes. Then sit on the toilet and push out. A second flushing this way will ensure all is clean and tidy up there.

Some will unscrew the shower head and place the open end of the flexible pipe against their anus. There's no need to insert it; the water pressure will instantly open your anus and let the water flow in. This really is a tricky operation and has many drawbacks.

First, you have no idea how much pressure is behind this forced jet of water and no idea how quickly it will deliver just half-a-pint. Unless you test for temperature first, you also risk being scalded or shocking the internal system with it being too cold. Too much water being forced in like this will continue its journey from the rectum on into the large intestine and further if you allow it. This has two undesirable effects.

With that much water inside you, you can expect it to trickle back down and out for quite awhile. It's awful to be expelling waste, no matter how thinned out it may be, while trying to enjoy your sexual games. Finally, although periodical irrigation, under medical supervision, may be okay, frequent enemas will wash away the natural and necessary inhabitants of your rectum, which can lead to problems of a different kind.

Back to the blog responses with Old Guy:

> *In the eye-ear care section of your pharmacy, you can buy an "Adult Ear Syringe" for about six bucks. It is intended for earwax control/cleansing, but works fine for the purposes discussed here. It holds three ounces and will do a nice job of "irrigating" the rectum. May require a couple of applications, but it works just fine.*

Respondent, Maria, says:

> *I think having an enema twice is the best idea, but don't get up from the toilet too fast. Make sure all the water and poop comes out. Once you're clean in and out, and you're ready, your partner will put some Vaseline on his fingers. Slowly, he starts massaging your rectum with one finger, then with two and finally with three, opening the hole slowly. Don't forget to kiss and do other things while he is doing that.*

> *By the time he is ready to introduce you, your hole is already dilated and slowly he gets in. Believe me it is not painful like that, and you will enjoy the experience. From that day forward, you will beg your partner to do you in the ass. I'm not kidding, do it like that.*

Easy Quick Clean! says:

> *Bath tip! Take a squeezey water bottle, fill it with lukewarm water to the top, squat over it, place tip inside your anus, and squeeze firmly. Hold it in and go to the toilet. Push the water out and repeat until satisfied following the same steps as above.*

> *This takes a matter of minutes and leaves a lovely clean bottom to be filled and dirtied up! Now use plenty of lube.*

These tips are for the men, too! You don't have to be gay to appreciate what I'm going to say here.

Men also have an abundance of nerve endings in and around the anus. They also have an erogenous zone that can ONLY be reached and stimulated via the entrance to the rectum: the prostate gland. The prostate gland produces so much of the seminal fluid and can be felt on the upper side of his rear passage (when he is lying on his back), by inserting a finger to about the second joint.

Blow his Mind

Using all the foregoing advice about preparation and relaxation, insert your finger with your palm upward until you can feel a smooth bulge. His prostate is roughly the size of a large walnut. Massage it gently, and you can make him cum this way—even without touching his penis! Do this while giving him a blow job or a hand-job, and you will blow his mind!

Here are some more thoughtful blog responses:

Stephanie says:

> *A boyfriend in college introduced me to anal sex. Until that time, I had only had oral and vaginal sex. He was good sized. However, after plenty of foreplay and lube, I found that it felt amazing—just very "full." Now that I'm married, I have anal sex with my husband, and I'm able to achieve an amazing orgasm if I stimulate my clitoris while having anal sex.*

Sarah says:

> *I am one of those women who prefer anal sex. It turns me on like no other form of sex. My current boyfriend is very well endowed, and I love the way he feels in me more than my average sized boyfriends. He hits spots I never knew existed!*

Bendover says:

> *While my wife and I both enjoy anal sex where I penetrate her, the best sex happens when she penetrates me. It took me years to get up the nerve to ask her to do me, but now we do it more often than any other sex act—her strap-on dildo is always erect, unlike my penis. I think a lot of guys who are penetrating their women are fantasizing about switching roles.*

Jena says:

> *Sex is an amazing thing in all its ways, but it's up to you on what you want to try. I have had anal sex with four guys and only enjoyed it with three of them.*

Mikkey says:

> *After three years of togetherness, my boyfriend and I tried anal sex. Truth be told, it was incredible. We tried once before, fairly early on in the relationship, but it was too painful (my partner's a big boy). However, recently I have enjoyed anal stimulation when having sex in doggie style and decided that perhaps I could try again. At no point did my partner pressure me. Lots of lube + Clit stimulator = Amazing!*

Jaycee says:

> *I enjoy anal play. Pain is not inevitable for the woman, if you a work into it by using fingers. Start with one first and work up to three. Use lots of lube. Breathe and relax.*
>
> *One way to really get into it is for the woman to squat or kneel over her man and very slowly lower herself onto shaft bit by bit, moving up and down in tiny increments. Her man*

may help "aim" but should not push until the woman is very relaxed and comfortable. In this position, the woman has more control of penetration, and by facing each other they can communicate easier, enjoy each others facial expressions, and have plenty of clitoral stimulation. Fantastic!!

An Honest Guy says:

I must say that more and more of my girlfriends are asking me for anal sex; some even expect it as part of our usual sexual routine. Being a caring sort of bloke, and having asked my girlfriends what their views on anal sex are, I get two answers:

1. *Depending on how the woman is built and her mood, anal sex heightens pleasure and gives a more intense experience.*

2. *It's a naughty girl fantasy/control thing . . . or just fun to do something seen as kinky or different.*

So, at the end of the day, as long as the two of you are honest about what you want and like and are caring, it's all good. THOUGH I WILL SAY . . . .

- *The more lube, the better.*

- *Guys be gentle; she must also be very relaxed and happy to play!*

- *Even more lube.*

- *Did I mention lube?*

Positions for Anal Sex

The two obvious positions for the woman are 'missionary position' lying on her back with her knees bent and apart and 'doggy style' with the woman on all fours, with her hands supporting her forward weight.

A third position that gives the woman more control is with the man lying on his back and the woman straddles across him, so she can guide his penis in to her anus and control the speed and the depth of his penetration. He can hold his penis upright to 'take aim.' This position is referred to as the 'cowgirl' when she faces forward. She can also face his feet, known as the 'reverse cowgirl.' Naturally, these are good positions for vaginal penetration but equally good for anal— but, only for advanced anal students. Begin with the missionary and doggy and build up toward the cowgirl.

For the first few times, use only your hands to massage and fingers to penetrate. Massage using plenty of lube, with the woman lying flat on her stomach, is the best way to initiate relaxation. Study massage techniques a little, so you can become more of an expert. Massage not only her back, neck and shoulders but also her arms and legs. Don't forget her hands and feet. Resist diving into her anus or vulva; that'll come later.

When she's content with her back massage, ask her to turn over and work on her front. Start, again at the top and work your way across her breasts and down her tummy and across her hips. Continue down her legs and gently move her legs apart as you do so, paying attention to her inner thighs. By this time, she will be anticipating your hands moving towards her vulva; don't disappoint her.

Place a pillow under her buttocks and use your fingers to relax her anus. Don't just dive in. Take your time and begin finger massaging the perineum, the point between her vagina and her anus, and work towards her anus.

Lube, lube, lube, and follow the tips given previously. No penis this time, or probably the next few times—just your fingers. Don't push your finger into her anus. Run the tip of your finger along the perineum and bring it to rest upon her anus, then gently apply more pressure to the tip and allow it to slip into her anus. No pumping action, just slowly continue to insert.

Talk to her while you're doing this and let her know how much you're enjoying it. Ask her if she would like to turn over and go doggy—style. She will then be in the very best position to give you full access and vision.

Follow the tips and continue to use just your fingers. Don't poke or prod. Always be gentle and use finger movements within the anus, like a figure of eight with your finger tip, to relax the muscles.

In either position, when you have a finger, or two as she becomes more relaxed, inserted as far as you can go into her anus, use your free hand to massage her vulva and stimulate her clitoris. If she shows signs of growing excitement, don't change the rhythm. Change now and she will lose the momentum. In other words, she is in control of directing her orgasm—you simply provide the stimulus.

It's exactly the same for her as it is for you when she's giving you a hand-job. You feel the climax building and know that if she continues the way she's doing it, you will orgasm. If she changes her rhythm or the way she's holding your penis, you suddenly lose that building climax. It's exactly the same for her when you start to get it right; don't change. No, there's no need to speed up, just keep what you're doing and she will explode!

Don't be afraid to experiment, but ALWAYS communicate. Tell her that she might find it easier or more stimulating if you enter her from another angle. Do nothing without her agreement. Be gentle. Be loving. Be adventurous.

The first time she invites you to replace your fingers with your penis, go really slow. More lube and no thrusting. Tell her to breathe deeply; this will help her continue her relaxation. Doggy is best, so you can hold onto her hips, but she does all the moving. This way you know how much she wants to accept. When she stops moving back onto you, use your hands to stimulate her clitoris and continue to wait for her to decide on anal movements.

Anal Sex and Safety

Anal sex should always be practiced with care, for both heterosexual and homosexual couples, to be as safe as possible. Condoms can help protect against a variety of health concerns. Also, both you and your partner should go in for STD screening prior to venturing into the anal sex arena, Here are some of the potential health risks.

- **Human Immunodeficiency Virus (HIV)**—Anal intercourse does come with the highest risk of contracting this disease than any other sexual activities.

- **Human Papiloma Virus (HPV)**—This virus can be passed via anal intercourse and can lead to anal warts or anal cancer.

- **Hepatitis A**—This infectious disease can be passed through oral-anal contact.

- **Hepatitis C**—This sometimes deadly liver disease is, in rare instances, passed via anal intercourse.

- **Urinary Tract Infection**—This, most-often, can occur when fecal matter comes into contact with the urethra of a woman. For this reason, always clean off your penis or fingers if your going to touch your partner's vagina after anal play.

- **Escherichia coli (E. coli)**—This bacterial disease can be passed with oral-anal contact, and is also one bacteria that can cause a urinary tract infection.

Again, always use a condom and water-based lubricant when having anal sex. There are even special, toughened condoms designed specifically for anal sex that may enhance protection.

Final Thoughts

I'm going to let Batwoman have the last word on anal sex:

As for anal sex, I can certainly believe that some women may never like it. That's a shame, but it really does require a lot of things to be in alignment—the right partner (perhaps very hard to come by), a willingness to be very open-minded about sex in general (perhaps also very hard to come by), lots of time, lots of lube, and lots of trust. That's a lot of things that have to go right all at the same time. If any one is missing, the lady is not going to enjoy the experience and may be scarred by it, so she will never enjoy it in the future, either.

I also think that some guys are just too big for anal sex to feel good for a woman. I have no experience over about 5.0 EG (erect girth), but my guess is that anything over 5.5 EG would be too much for me to enjoy anally.

It can come as a major surprise (if you are an adult) to discover that there really are new things about sex that you can learn. It is really very much worth taking the time and trouble!

Some folks use enemas (squirt water inside the rectum to clean everything out first), but I have never done that. I just try to make sure I "go" hours before hand and clean up well. A warm washcloth is never amiss.

As for getting faeces on things, this is not a big problem. The guy will of course want to wash afterward, and there may be smudges on his cock afterward, but usually not much. Many folks who engage in anal use condoms for just that reason. If you have anal sex unprotected, you can get some brownish stains on the bed sheets afterward, especially if you cum inside your partner. Don't be surprised or grossed out—it is all natural and just part of how bodies work.

For health reasons, being careful with hygiene is important. Washing well, using condoms, only engaging in anal with partners you know really well and trust—those are key. I would also add that a guy should NEVER insert his cock in his partner's pussy after anal, unless he has washed first or replaced whatever condom he used in her ass. A lady DOES NOT need extra bacteria from anal pushed into her vagina!

You may see scenes in porn in which a guy goes straight from anal into the mouth of his partner. I would never want to do that. My guess is that the ladies in those shots did a huge amount of enema work beforehand to make sure they were absolutely totally clean inside before starting. And they got paid a lot of money for it!

I don't think that a curved penis* would matter at all.

Everything inside her is flexible and moveable; the main obstacle is getting past the rings of muscle at the entrance. A curve will have no effect on that part.

For anal sex to be enjoyable for her, the most important things are for you to be well-lubed and patient (both critical), and for her to relax enough to take you and enjoy it. If you go slowly and take your time with anal play before trying full penetration, you should be fine.

You should also know that a lady does not have complete control over what her ass does. She may want to relax, but if the body isn't ready, it just isn't. She has to be patient with herself, too, and work with you to make her ready. I found that a bit hard to learn at first, since my vagina opens (more or less) when I want it to. I was surprised/frustrated that I could not make my anus do the same thing. I had to learn to cede control and let my partner (and my ass!) figure out when I was really ready for him. This has gotten a lot easier with time and practice.

*Note: Most men have a slight twist in their penis. Some are more pronounced than others. This is known as 'penile torsion.' This is because the human body is made from two halves, which develop at slightly different rates before birth. Interestingly, the twist is always anti—clockwise.

── 19 ──

Masturbation

Don't knock masturbation. It's sex with someone you love.

~ Woody Allen

"Masturbation"—some think of it as a dirty word. I'd like to dispel the notion masturbation is dirty, unnecessary, or women never do it.

I've read surveys that show 98 percent of men masturbate, and 68 percent of women masturbate as well. Where they get these figures from, I do not know, but I have a sneaky feeling very, very few people of either sex do not masturbate on a regular basis.

My friend, Batwoman, may be exceptional, but her view on masturbation is worth reading.

> *I have no idea why masturbation is ever thought of in a negative light. It is in no way dirty, sick, or perverted. It is totally natural, something we are designed to do. How can there be anything wrong with something that feels so good and hurts nobody?*
>
> *I think everybody masturbates—certainly all men and probably most women. I do. My partner does, and we both*

enjoy talking about it and doing it for each other (both remotely and in front of each other).

Shared Intimacy

Batwoman continues discussing the benefits of masturbation and shared intimacy.

I love the shared intimacy, and I think there is nothing hotter than watching a guy stroke himself, or hearing about it from him after the fact. However, it is indeed a very intimate act.

In my younger years, I never admitted to anyone that I masturbated. I never asked a man if he did. I think it's due to social conditioning, plus the fact it is a profoundly personal act. When you admit such very personal things to another person, you are inviting them inside you in a way that can make you feel vulnerable. That feels good with somebody you really trust, but maybe not so good if you are unsure of yourself.

I certainly did not feel badly when my man told me about his masturbation. He's a man; I knew he did it. I was just glad he was willing to talk about it with me. However, I am a totally grown up woman, and we were very close before we started talking about such things. My advice, if you want to start talking to a girl about this—go slowly.

Mutual Masturbation

When you are comfortable with the fact both of you enjoy the feeling masturbation brings, it can become part of foreplay. Not with yourself, but to and with your partner. This is a particularly enjoyable part of foreplay, for those in advancing years (or not so supple backs). Of course, this is not to say it can't be practiced at any age!

With both of you lying side-by-side, reach out with the hand nearest to each other's genitals. The first time you do this, let your partner guide you with their free hand over yours. This way the girl can stroke the man's penis the way he likes it, and the man will be shown the best way to stimulate her clitoris and labia.

Relax and take your time. You will sense when your partner is ready to speed up, slow down or move to the next position.

Remote Mutual Masturbation—or Virtual Sex

Thanks to improvements in technology, remote virtual masturbation, AKA virtual sex, is now not just an erotic idea of science—fiction writers. This is especially valuable for couples who have to spend time apart due to travel schedules for work, living in different areas or because they are military stationed overseas. A whole new industry is emerging—teledildonics.

Companies like Remote Pleasure and Mojowijo offer vibration masturbators your partner can control no matter where they're located geographically. For the Mojowijo, there is both a male and a female masturbator. The female masturbator is a dildo and the male masturbator features a circular c-shaped device that goes around the penis shaft. Each partner controls the intensity of the the other person's masturbator. Using Skype and a webcam, it takes virtual sex a step closer to the real thing than ever before.

Both Remote Pleasure and Mojowijo devices are easy to use. Software is downloaded by both partners and all that is needed is an Internet connection. It's an entirely new way to stay connected with your partner, even when you can't physically be with them. Better than sexting, with teledildonics you can now not only see your partner, but control what they feel.

Although nothing can replace having your partner right there with you, teledildonics can be the next best thing. It may even help curb a person's temptation to stray while apart from their partner. Plus, this is only the beginning, with teledildonics really only taking off in 2012. Surely, the technology will continue to advance, especially with the growing number of long-distance relationships.

Alternative Method of Female Masturbation

Many women masturbate using their index finger to stimulate their clitoris. However, there is another way to masturbate women may like to try. This method not only gives a lot of pleasure, but it also exercises your PC muscle at the same time.

Remember I said to exercise your 'love muscle' as frequently as possible? Well, here's a time when it's going to give you enjoyment and even an orgasm!

Pinch your clitoris between your finger and thumb. If you're like many women, your clitoris is well hidden and not very big. If this is the case, you might have to use your fingers to start the blood flowing into this area, just as you would have done before with masturbation, in order to engorge your clit enough to be able to pinch it. Now, when I say "pinch the clitoris," I don't mean pull it right out there, free of its hood. Just pinch your clit, hood and all.

Hold the pinch and Kegel. Feel your clit swell a little with each Kegel. Continue Kegeling and with each squeeze of your PC muscle your clitoris will engorge with more blood. After awhile you'll hold the hood and your clit will slide up and down between finger and thumb with each Kegel. This action is identical to a man when he holds his penis and his foreskin rolls back and forth over his glans.

Enjoy!

——— 20 ———

Pornography

Pornography is the quadraphonics of sex.

It adds a third and fourth track to the sexual act.

~ Jean Baudrillard

It's Only Natural

Men and women have a natural curiosity about each other's bodies and bodily functions. Inquiring minds find it difficult to ignore an opportunity to see a naked body when it presents itself. No matter how pure of mind you might be, if a naked person suddenly appeared in your line of vision, most of us would be tempted to peek beyond looking into their eyes, even if only for a moment.

It is only natural for your gaze to drop to the genitals of another naked person. How long does this 'viewing' have to be taken before it becomes unnatural or even obsessive?

I have written before, in order to reassure men who expressed a concern about finding themselves looking at other naked males in the changing rooms or showers at the gym, about how this is a completely natural reaction. In no way does it suggest they are becoming gay.

Women too find themselves comparing their own bodies with other girls in the changing rooms, and the same rule applies. It is only when a glance becomes a constant interest, and is taken further by expressing an interest to the object (person) of your desire, when a question about your sexual orientation might arise.

History of Pornography

Cavemen carved simple pictures of couples copulating on the walls of their home, alongside pictures of all the other activities they were involved in during their days. We can't imagine seeing a couple of stick—people etched into a cave wall making us ready for love-making nowadays—although it might plant the mental suggestion.

Explicit painting of various sexual positions were discovered in the brothels of ancient Pompeii, detailing the services provided. In ancient Greece, depictions of sexual positions were found at the bottom of children's plates, so they had something entertaining to look at when they finished eating their meal. In Athens, the phallic statues of Priapus were placed on street corners, so women could come and pray in front of them for fertility.[114]

Pornography as a general depiction of the human form and/or the act of copulation, is as old as mankind itself. As we have progressed technically through the ages, statues of all kinds of creatures, including the naked male and female form were hewn from rock and wood and metal. When printing came into existence, it gave pornography a new medium to utilize, plus allowed for increased opportunities for mobility and distribution.

Print

The Greeks have a word for it—*pornographos*. Translated, this means 'writing about prostitutes.' Here we have a clue to what activities readers hoped to read about—sexually titillating material.

Add a few pictures and we have the beginnings of recognizable pornography in still form.

The *Kama Sutra*, the ancient Indian treatise on rules governing physical relationship, love and marriage, was compiled in the 3rd century by Vatsyayana. Complete with erotic illustrations depicting the sexual knowledge of ages past, the central belief of the *Kama Sutra* is in order for a couple to have a happy marriage, both partners must be well-versed in the art of both carnal and cerebral pleasure. This is the oldest known book on sensual pleasures.

Modern print pornography, however, saw its beginnings in 16th century Rome, thanks to the Italian Renaissance. In 1524, Marcantonio Raimondi published 16 sexually explicit engravings, designed by Giulio Romano. Titled the *I Modi,* figures from Greco-Roman mythology to Classical antiquity were depicted enjoying carnal pleasures. The engravings caused quite a scandal and Pope Clement VIII imprisoned Raimondi for nearly a year, until a consortium negotiated his release.[115]

This consortium included Pietro Aretino. This Italian author, satirist and polemicist is often referred to as the father of modern pornography. He authored two pornographic masterpieces—*Sonetti Lussuriosi*, in 1527, and *Ragionamenti* in 1534. *Sonetti Lussuriosi* featured sexually explicit sonnets that were illustrated with Romano's images from *I Modi. Ragionamenti* was a continuation of Aretino's work, in the form of a dialogue between two prostitutes. Both were highly popular with the aristocracy of the Renaissance Age.[116]

In the 18th century, *Memoirs of a Woman of Pleasure*, also known as *Fanny Hill,* was written by John Cleveland and published between 1748 and 1749. This was the first English prose-based pornography and the first pornographic novel. The novel was determined to be so obscene, it remained 'underground' until the mid-1960s, when it became popularly printed in the United States.[117]

Although printing technology helped facilitate the distribution of pornography, it was still only available to those who knew where to find it and could afford to pay for it. However, as time passed, its distribution became more widespread and included the advent of 'gentleman's' magazines. As the 20th century approached, magazines such as *Le Frisson, Nickell* and *Metropolitan* became popular. In the US in the 1920s, the *Tijuana Bibles* were published, featuring erotic comics, dirty stories, and pin-up girls. The addition of color resulted in an explosion of interest, yet you still had to pay for it, and in December 1953 Hugh Hefner published the first edition of *Playboy Magazine*, including a nude Marilyn Monroe as the iconic magazine's first centerfold.[118]

Film

Even before television was invented, black and white moving films were made illicitly of copulating couples for distribution to 'dirty old men,' as perceived by the general populace. From 1896 to 1970, stag films were illegal movies often smuggled in for bachelor parties and college fraternities. Stag films of the early 20th century were often silent and short (less than 15 minutes long). These black and white films were most often crude amateur videos with disjointed narratives.[119]

In the late 1960s and early 1970s, Sweden's Lasse Braun revolutionized the pornographic film industry. Using high quality, color Super 8mm (and later 16mm) film, Braun made 80 color films, ranging in length from eight to 15 minutes each. These were shot in exotic locations and had a variety of plot lines, from spy thrillers to historical dramas.[120]

Today, the pornographic film industry is booming. A new movie is being made every 39 minutes, in the United States.[121] Full-length and semi-full length films may include not only complex story lines (including spoofs of popular movies), but also intricate costuming, sets and even special effects. The digital age now sees films recorded and distributed widely, so viewers can enjoy them in the privacy of their own home, at their leisure, as often as they'd like.

The Internet

Over the last couple of decades, the number of web pages with sexual content has grown from a few only the most determined and deliberate search would find, to a truly global phenomenon. In 2011, Google statistics indicated more than 755 million pages with sexual content. The global internet porn industry is worth $97 billion (£60 billion) a year. The second most expensive website name is sex.com, which cost $13 million (£8 million).[122]

Around 11,000 pornographic films are made each year in the US—ten times more than mainstream Hollywood movies. Most are for use on the World Wide Web.[123]

Driven by money, this industry often targets the simplest market: the testosterone-fueled male mind seeking visual stimulation aimed at sexual release through watching his chosen fantasies, without having to leave the privacy of his room or engaging with any other person. However, despite common disbelief, women too are enjoy pornography.

Women and Pornography

Although women may not want to admit to their family and friends their enjoyment of pornography, the reality is they are at least as stimulated by pornography as men. Theresa Flynt, vice president of marketing for Hustler Video, notes women account for 56 percent of their company's business at video stores. As she told CNN, "And, the female audience is increasing. (. . .) Women are buying more porn."[124]

Additionally, women are creating more pornography. Female director, Candida Royalle, makes hard-core, erotic videos specifically for female viewers. These sell at a rate of 10,000 copies per month![125]

In March 2010, the UK had its first female director of adult films selected as a Liberal Democratic parliamentary candidate.

Anna Arrowsmith, managing director of the Easy on the Eye film company, stood for the party in Gravesend, Kent, England. However, she failed to get elected. Under the name Anna Span, she has produced approximately 300 pornographic films, specializing in "women-friendly" titles such as *Where's the Rent Boys?* aimed at female erotica enthusiasts. She was named best director in the 2008 and 2009 UK Adult Film and Television Awards.[126]

Although society may wish to think it's only pervy, socially-inept men visiting pornographic websites, women are also increasingly checking out porn sites. A study by Family Safe Media found:

- 1 out of every 3 visitors to adult websites were female,

- 13 percent of women admit to accessing pornography at work, and

- 17 percent of women admit to struggling with pornography addiction.[127]

Men and women are physiologically very similar to one another, when it comes to their response to pornographic material. A 2006 study, conducted at McGill University, monitored the genital temperature of volunteers, to measure sexual arousal while viewing pornography. Both men and women began to display signs of arousal within 30 seconds. Men reached their maximum arousal level in 11 minutes. Women reached their maximum arousal level in 12 minutes. According to the researchers of the study, this is a statistically negligible difference.[128]

Hooked

In the beginning of the Internet pornography boon, you had to pay to enter these x-rated websites, before you were shown anything other than some soft porn still pictures. Now, with competition so fierce, most websites allow free viewing of full-blown porn as 'samples' of what you can expect to see more of with your purchase.

With such proliferation, many people who would not have chosen to view porn have had porn thrust upon them with spam e-mails. These unsolicited, electronic advertisements often end up in the person's trash folder, or even never reach the user thanks to improving spam filters. However, as in fishing, if the porn purveyors spread their nets wide enough, they catch a surprising number and variety of folk the porn websites would never have dreamed of approaching under normal circumstances. Growing numbers have been caught in the net and hooked by the bait.

Figures published in 2011 show pornography was viewed by 35.9 percent of Internet users in the UK. Broken down by gender, 44.3 percent of all men and 23.4 percent of all women who used the Internet looked at adult material.[129]

In the United States, every second:

- $3,075.64 is spent on pornography,

- 28.258 Internet viewers are viewing pornography and

- 372 Internet users are typing adult search terms into search engines.[130]

And those figures don't take into account the vast amount of pornographic material spread through chat rooms, message boards, so—called dating sites and shared images. Concerns regarding desensitization are real. Expose a person to enough of a certain type of material and it becomes normal.

The Generation, Cultural and Gender Gap

Pornography affects different people in different ways, and much of this has to do with the ideals and societal norms of different generations or different cultures. Those in their 50s, 60s and older, who grew up in a time where pornographic films were still illegal and may be more reticent concerning pornography. However, it can be helpful in discovering aspects of sex they never knew before. Pornography can add spice and renewed interest to their sex lives. However, it is important they share their new desires with their partners. One of the primary dangers of pornography occurs when one partner finds solace in porn that isolates them from their partner. This can significantly damage a relation, and can even end in divorce!

Culturally, the acceptance of pornography varies widely. Although Western society has, for the most part, legalized pornography, other cultures have not. In countries such as India and Russia, pornography is only legal with significant restrictions. Middle Eastern, a handful of Eastern European countries and China have a pornography ban. Despite the global pervasiveness of the Internet, countries such as Egypt are striving to force a more conservative culture on their citizens ordering a ban on online pornography.[131]

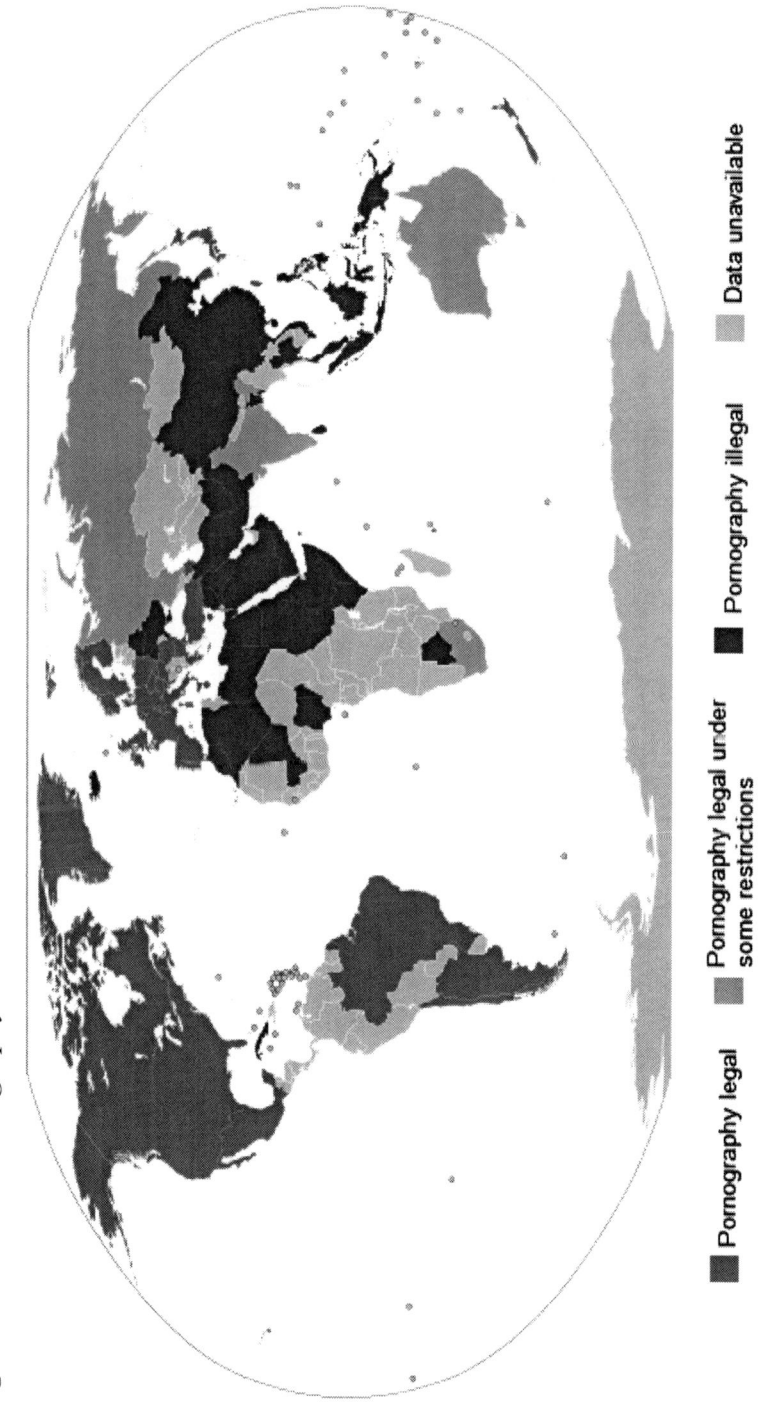

Figure 18: Global Pornography Laws [132]

Pornography legal
Pornography legal under some restrictions
Pornography illegal
Data unavailable

Even more open-minded, free-thinking countries struggle internally with the pornography question. Concerns over morality and the objectifying of women in porn arise in even the United States and UK. Most-often backed by religious organizations, these concerned citizens worry about the negative effects of pornography on individuals as well as society as a whole. Children advocates also have a strong voice, concerned with the long-term psychological effects of childhood exposure to pornography.

In addition to generational and cultural differences in the acceptance of pornography, there is also a fundamental difference between men and women. For men, sex is a biological imperative to procreate. Given the opportunity, a man will get an erection and fuck whoever is offering sex, and (barring any problems) the act will bring him to orgasm.

Men's thoughts are easily turned to sex when glimpsing a pretty face, a deep cleavage or pert bottom—even a sensuous image on an advertising poster. There's no getting away from it, and modern man has had to learn to control his lustful impulses in this civilized world, in order to fit in with society. Within a monogamous relationship, neither partner is expected to wander, nor do they wish to if the bond of love is present.

The attraction of porn is it immediately frees a person from all constraints, and they can satisfy their lusty fantasies whenever they want. When porn is used incorrectly, there is no need to look for a partner and no need to learn about human interactions. In its most alienating form, there is no need to express to a partner the person's deepest or darkest desires and no need for respect or the time to get to know someone. There is just instant physical gratification. Sad but true.

One Woman's Perspective

by Kimberly Wylie

As Clive has pointed out throughout this book, we're all different. For this reason, I preface my addition here with the disclaimer—this is my personal perspective, as well as what I know from my immediate circle of friends. I think the key to any healthy relationship is communication. As with all things intimate, discussing preferences with your partner in a respectful and caring manner is critical.

With this said, whether we want to admit it or not, many women enjoy pornography. Although sometimes it may be sappy, romantic porn, where there are two people in a loving relationship we want to watch, it also can be completely based on fantasy—something completely unlike what we have in real life, things that even go beyond our personal fantasies, to more lurid imaginings. The reality is, pornography holds the same titillation factor for women as it does for men.

Yup, women can be just as perverted as men!

In fact, oftentimes we'd rather pornography not be about a caring, loving relationship. Chances are, we have this at home. This would be akin to watching a television program about a mom uneventfully cleaning the house, driving the kids to soccer practice and then coming home to make dinner. Boring!!

Take a simple look at the popularity of the *50 Shades of Grey* series or the *Sookie Stackhouse* novels (and their incredibly casted HBO series—*True Blood*) or even the movie *Magic Mike*. Like men, women enjoy fantasizing and exploring their sensuality. The question then becomes—Why do women sometimes seem to have a problem with pornography?

There are five core reasons why a woman may have an issue with porn.

- Societal norms still affect what is "acceptable" for women. We may have come along way, baby, in the last century, but the reality is there is not full gender equality in our world. This isn't necessarily a bad thing in all cases, but when it comes to women and sex/desiring sex/being sexual, this antiquated attitude can be detrimental to a woman's inner sexual goddess.

- Men's use of pornography detracting from a relationship. If a man is spending time alone with pornography instead of having intimate relations with his woman, it's no wonder these women feel negatively about porn!

- Concerns regarding body image. Although there is an increasing amount of porn out there depicting a variety of body sizes and shapes, the majority still features young, nubile women with perfect (although often surgically-altered) breasts, flat stomachs and not a stretch mark upon them. That can be intimidating—especially to those of us who've had a few more decades on them, plus a couple of kids! The important thing here is to make sure your woman knows and feels how beautiful you think she is!

- Pornography addiction negatively affecting a couple's sex life. This goes beyond simply a reduction in sex, due to a man's use of masturbation and pornography, but the other negative effects that can occur with addiction, such as the man's inability to have sex without the use of pornography or the unrealistic expectations he may have of his partner, spurred by pornography.

- Unpalatable pornography making a woman uncomfortable. Most people have scenes/acts they simply don't find a turn-on. Of course, this is true of men as well as women.

In the end, many women will agree pornography can be a fun occasional addition to an active and exciting sex life. It can give you new ideas of positions to try or toys to use, or simply ramp up the excitement! In fact, my husband and I sometimes treat porn like Mystery Science Theater, making fun of the really, really bad ones. What better way to spend the evening with your lover—laughing and turned on!

Just remember—communication, communication, communication!

Respect your woman's boundaries and ideas. Make her feel loved, wanted and cherished and never, ever use pornography as a substitute for being with her.

Pornography and the Birds and the Bees

If you were born into the current generation, which has never been without the Internet, viewing porn may have been the easy option when your inquisitive mind wanted to learn about sex—or so you may have thought. Instead of asking a parent or referring to some other responsible professional source of educated wisdom, you may have avoided the embarrassment of displaying ignorance and feeling a fool among your peers.

In some instances, especially when a young person's parents are unwilling or unable to effectively communicate the information regarding the birds and the bees, the Internet can be a sexual resource. Only a couple of generations ago sexual myths, such as getting pregnant from a toilet seat, were common among uneducated teens. Although exposure to pornography as a developing teenager has significant concerns, is it more disturbing than the young woman who only finds out the true mechanics of sex on her wedding night?

This is where parents need to take responsibility for their children and their sexual education. Parents need to instill morality in their child, not allow it to be at the whims of society. Teaching children about the value of loving, respectful relationships is key to developing the stability of the next generation. It's also important to not only monitor a child's Internet activity, but also to warn them about the dangers of pornography addiction, just as you would any other substance addiction concern.

I read a letter from an exasperated, not to say sadly disappointed, woman who spoke of a former partner who had watched porn on the Internet from his formative teenage years. Now aged 31, she said he was incapable of a normal sexual relationship and has had this problem all his sexual life. She said, "We were very much in love, but he had a problem with sex. He was so acclimatized to porn, sex in a relationship was almost incomprehensible to him." Porn was like a drug to him; he could not get or keep an erection without using porn.

Age of Innocence

Before the Internet, pubescent kids and young adults would sneak a peek at pictures of partially dressed girls in men's magazines. By today's standards both the pictures and the kids were total innocents. They had to grow up and discover the joys of intimacy through learning self-control, communication, expressing feelings and desire without offending. This situation provided fertile ground for making friends and bonding through common interests and, yes, some rejection, too. It also created opportunities for nurturing true love, maybe borne out of lust to begin with but developing into lasting relationships. Thankfully this can still happen, but all too frequently is spoiled due to exposure to pornography.

Body changes can be frightening and confusing in the minds of children who have no idea what is happening to them. An erection is the subject of curiosity to a seven-year old boy but waking up to his first nocturnal emission can be, at best, disconcerting and, at worst, impregnate his mind with the thought he is somehow dirty and needs to hide his guilty secret.

The answer to these scenarios is, of course, education. By whom, and at what age? It is a dilemma constantly confronting educationalists but, in my estimation, always best done by a loving parent, preferably a joint exercise between a mother and father. These are the only people close enough to see the signs coming along and judging the right time (physically and mentally) for their offspring—no two are the same!

If you are a parent, there are parental controls you can apply to your kids computers and mobile devices. However, there is nothing you can substitute for your personal monitoring of your children and their Internet activities, as well as the discussions you have with your kids regarding sexual relationships and what you feel is acceptable concerning the topic of pornography.

Again, easy access to pornography, whether it be dad's *Playboy*, the soft-core pornography featured on cable channels such as Showtime, or the ever-growing supply of pornography via the Internet, means parents have to be proactive in their child's sexual education. Exposure to pornography can warp a child's mind about what sex is and how people should act. It can lead to a desensitization to the act itself. As with the pervasiveness of drugs in today's society, a parent's communication with their child about what is and is not appropriate, and acknowledgment of the related dangers, is key to ensuring your child develops into a healthy sexual being, who understands pornography is not for everyone. However, for those interested in it, between two consenting adults and used as a complement to a respectful, sexual relationship, it can add spice to a couple's life.

The Dangers of Pornography

As mentioned, there are both generational, cultural and gender differences that factor into whether a person finds pornography acceptable and to what degree. It would be too easy to ignore the differences and simply describe the possible dangerous effects of porn to be applicable to 'impressionable' people only. The saddest reality is this description has to be applied to the youngest group shown above.

Without careful parental communication and education, children can be exposed to pornographic material and think this is what love and sex is all about—and how grown-ups behave. Late in 2012, allegedly a case of rape was brought against a ten-year old boy in the UK. In this unconfirmed case reported in a UK national newspaper, he repeatedly raped his 12-year old next door neighbor girl, over a period of two months. He sometimes even invited his friends to watch. The boy was reported as saying he just wanted to be 'grown-up.' Unfortunately, the numbers of such cases are growing and, in the UK especially, there is a groundswell movement by parents who want to see a block on internet porn in the UK. This movement was widely reported by the media and featured women behind the website www.mumsnet.com.

Addicted to Porn

Pornography addiction is a very real problem, due to the chemical responses to sexual stimulation to the brain. Nature has ensured we continue to perform activities that are critical to our survival—eating and having sex. As a reward to these species-survival activities, the brain is programmed to release dopamine—a feel-good chemical that encourages us to repeat this behavior. Like sex with another person, viewing pornography causes a very similar increase in dopamine levels; however the levels remain elevated for a longer period of time than sex, giving an increased sensation of reward.[133] For some, this dopamine high through porn becomes preferred to actual sex with another person. This is when pornography addiction begins.

Following are 5 signs you may have a porn addiction problem:

1. You have an increasing amount of computer memory or bookmarked websites devoted to pornography.

2. You view pornographic materials in inappropriate places, such as: the office, a coffee shop, school, etc.

3. You are spending an increasing amount of time masturbating with pornography rather than having sex with your partner.

4. You keep your pornographic viewing habits secret from your partner or lie about the extent of your pornographic viewing and/or masturbation.

5. You increasingly prefer solitude, missing opportunities to interact with real-life people, where you'd rather spend your time with porn.

If you're concerned you or a partner may be addicted to pornography, there are numerous addiction professionals who can provide you with additional information and assistance.

The Constantly Changing Face of Internet Pornography

Pornography on the internet is constantly changing. Although I mention YouPorn.com in my book, which is one of the largest websites for porn, new web pages are appearing all the time. Some sites may still be around and have similar content when you read this, as when I visited them while writing this book. Others may have changed. The examples I give here won't necessarily be around, or they may have evolved into something different by the time you read this book.

One website that differs substantially from YouPorn.com and other pornographic websites, and a site you may not normally think of as "pornographic," is http://sexisfashion.tumblr.com/. Tumblr allows users to share almost anything, including text, photos, quotes, links, music, and videos. Their tagline "Follow the world's creators." sums up perfectly the concept behind this popular site—a website where creative people can share their work with the world. Although it may have not been planned, this includes pornographic material.

At Tumblr, there are no advertisements but simply still photographs and short rolling-videos submitted by viewers. A list of reviewers who have left comments for you to see is shown with their user names—you can click on any icon and it will take you straight to pictures and videos collected and shown, by the reviewer. There is something to satisfy all inquiring minds. New material is added almost daily, so it is constantly changing.

It could be argued this type of pornography is more 'erotic' than pornographic, with many items works of art. Also the standard of photography is often far better than what you will see on YouPorn.com (and is not such a shock to the system when you first see it), it allows you to scroll through the pictures as you wish. Many Tumblr photos are of a professional studio standard, which would be suitable for any glossy magazine. However, you must be prepared to see sex acts in all their most intimate detail.

An interesting question to ask yourself when viewing these pornographic web pages is "Why?" Why did the people in the videos or photos agree to have themselves photographed or videoed, to be published on the Internet for the entire world to see, forevermore? Most importantly, if you're considering having pornographic photographs or videos of yourself published on the Internet, ask yourself, "Is this something I'd be embarrassed if my family saw it?" "Is this something I'd be embarrassed if my children or grandchildren saw it?" Think carefully, because once this material is published on the Internet, it is impossible to unring the bell.

Satisfy Your Curiosity

The difference between pornography and erotica is lighting.

~ Gloria Leonard

There is no doubt watching porn is titillating for both sexes. Additionally, it can be an invaluable tool in satisfying your curiosity about certain activities. There are even websites that claim to be educational. These sites can be excellent places to learn about new things you may want to try with your partner—answering questions about the logistics you may have. However, don't forget, sometimes porn actors have to take up unnatural positions to allow the camera to see what's happening.

Although there are a plethora of pay-to-view pornography sites, nowadays there is little reason to pay. There is such a choice of free material, from amateur to professional, even cartoon style (in 3D if you wish). It's a bit of a jungle for you to hack through. From heterosexual to gay, solo to lesbian, Caucasian to Asian, multiple partners to double—penetration, blow-jobs to cum-shots, the list is endless and constantly building. There are websites that even specialize in specific fetishes. The amount of variety can be mind boggling. With comprehensive free sites, like YouPorn.com, it does mean pornography isn't just easy to access, it's free.

Watch together —understanding what to expect from each other only enhances the experience. Anticipation builds sexual excitement. Make it fun and enjoy it!

Dealing with Addiction?

If you think you or your partner may be obsessed or addicted to pornography, where you or they can't do without it, you're not alone.

Thankfully, there is hope. There are many people who have become addicted to porn and have found ways to overcome the addiction. Here are a couple of websites set up by recovered porn addicts, describing how they did it:

- www.thelaughingmonkey.org
- www.feedtherightwolf.org

There are also a wide variety of psychological professionals who can assist you or your partner, should you feel pornography has become a negative force in your life. Never hesitate to seek professional help.

──── 21 ────

Fetish and Fantasy

I have a high-heel fetish. I love really beautiful women's
shoes. To me, it's not weird. I can take it all.

~ David Arquette

Are Fetishes Normal?

With the understanding of what fetish is, I think it's important to discuss it further. First, know most of us have a fetish. Sometimes we're not consciously aware of our fetishes. It's perfectly normal to be extra excited about something that may not excite your friends too much. Of course, maybe they're keeping their own thoughts to themselves.

There are times when you don't even have to be close to the 'thing' that turns you on. Just a thought, and it can become part of your fantasy. This is normal.

Parts of the body feature commonly in fetishes. This can even include particular shapes or color of body parts. Breasts feature strongly in most male fetishes or fantasies. Eyes, or even eyebrows, can make a girl melt with desire. Legs, feet, arms, navels, nipples, and noses—everyone has their particular favorite.

Paraphilia

According to *Psychology Today,* "A paraphilia (commonly known as a fetish) is a condition in which a person's sexual arousal and gratification depend on fantasizing about and engaging in sexual behavior that is atypical and extreme."[134] This fascination can focus on an object or on a particular act. Some paraphilias are more common in one sex than another. This focus for the person typically is very specific and doesn't change over time. This paraphilia can become such a preoccupation the person becomes dependent on the object or behavior to be sexually gratified.

Anil Aggrawal wrote extensively on the subject of paraphilias, the technical description of fetishes and compiled a list of 547 terms describing paraphilic sexual interests.[135]

547 . . . yup, this number astonished me too!

However, when you read his list which includes everything from necrophilia (sexual interest in corpses) to zoophilia (sexual interest in animals), you realize his list is really quite comprehensive. You may have to read hundreds of listings before you find a fetish that may apply to you.

Professor Aggrawal states in his book, "Not all these paraphilias have necessarily been seen in clinical setups. This may not be because they do not exist, but because they are so innocuous they are never brought to the notice of clinicians. Like allergies, sexual arousal may occur from anything under the sun, including the sun."

Mine? Well, I claim the right to keep that a secret! However, like most people, I do have one, and when I get close it drives my excitement into top gear!

By all means, talk about your fetishes with your partner. However, sharing them with others should be handled more cautiously. Also, sharing your personal fetishes on publicly-accessible websites, like social media, definitely should be given careful consideration. Once you place something on the Internet, it can never truly be deleted. Plus, more and more employers are searching social media websites to research potential candidates for open positions. It would be a shame to lose out on a career opportunity because you were too open with the Internet world with your particular fetishes.

Imagination

It doesn't matter what you do in the bedroom as long as you don't do it in the street and frighten the horses.

~ Mrs. Patrick Campbell

It's a short step from fetish to fantasy. Imagining oneself in certain situations might be out of your normal routine or with a person or persons unavailable to you (a film star or even a neighbor) are common elements of fantasy. Because sex has a mental component, fantasizing can bring you to a climax when all else is failing.

Men and women fantasize more often than they would care to admit. Fantasy is anything that gets you more excited than usual. Fantasy can be enriched even further by making use of a fetish. Your fantasy is driven and only limited by your imagination.

Using the Excitement of Fetish & Fantasy

There are certain sexual experiences that are more exciting than others. As an example, the first time you have sex with a partner, the newness and anticipation that built up to it can be so exciting it's indelibly etched in your memory. You can draw upon the memories of these extra-exciting experiences to increase the level of excitement, through fantasy, time and time again.

If you feel a rush of excitement with just the thought of having sex in a public place, for an example, with the risk of being caught pumping your adrenaline through the roof, this is putting a fantasy to the test. Sex in the open air, incidentally, is always rather special but best done somewhere you are confident you are not going to get caught or be watched.

Voyeurism (watching others in intimate situations) is another common fetish aspect born out of a mix of desire and fantasy. It's also another reason porn is so successful on the net—nobody knows you're watching! On the other side of this fetish equation, some fantasize about being watched. Some even deliberately leave the curtains open, to add the thrill of possibly having others watch.

Dressing up can mix fetish and fantasy. Do you remember playing "doctor" when we were kids? It's fun and can be liberating to act out scenarios and play dress-up, to pretend to be someone you're not. As adults, the fun can turn into sexual excitement, especially as inhibitions are removed through the character or costume. Uniforms can be fun and titlating—from a nurse to a waitress, policeman to sailor. Whether it's seamed stockings, masks, or other costumes, who knows what makes us desire such things. The important thing is to discuss your fantasies and fetishes with your partner and find a common ground to have them enhance your sex life.

The list is endless, and if you'd like to read what others get up to, or even join in on the discussions, you can find a free forum here—http://www.FetLife.com. FetLife describes itself as a "BDSM & fetish community for kinksters by kinksters."

Of course, as we indulge ourselves in these extra-curricular sexual activities, for some it's only a short step from fetish and fantasy to develop into something more serious—and possibly dangerous.

Eroticism

Feeling the need to pee on a long journey, the woman's boyfriend pulls the car over so she can relieve herself by the roadside bushes. She pulls down her jeans and squats over the grass. Although he can only just see her from where he's parked the car, he can clearly see her urine streaming from between her thighs and pouring into the soil. As the man watches, he can feel an erection coming on.

I'm telling you this story because it illustrates how easily one event can excite and interest a person to the point of wanting to investigate further. Something mundane can become erotic. Just as we're all different, our fantasies and fetishes are equally as different.

Examples of Fetishes

Water Sports

Also known as "Golden Showers," urolagnia is urinating, particularly in public, on others and/or being urinated on. Getting back to our two traveling companions, for some, warm pee splashed onto a naked body can be very erotic. Of course, don't do this unless both of you agree to try it.

With the woman lying in the bathtub, her man might stand alongside the tub and aim his pee at her clit. If you've never done this, you'll be amazed how powerful a light stream hitting this spot can be.

Outside, (no need to spend time laying out waterproofs) the man can lie on his back while his woman squats across his body and pees. She can work her way up toward his face. Don't worry. Urine, although different, doesn't taste that bad. Always spit it out, however. Guys, also never pee inside her vagina, and both of you should avoid peeing into the eyes.

Tip: Light colored urine is fine. Darker colored urine is an indicator of dehydration and tastes much stronger. Eat a healthy diet. You taste of what you eat and drink.

Spanking and Pain

Pain—known as Algolagnia, particularly involves an erogenous zone. It differs from masochism as there is a biologically different interpretation of the sensation, rather than a subjective interpretation. This is another practice that can escalate. It can start with light spanking across the buttocks (a fetish for buttocks, incidentally, is known as pygophilia). No real pain here, just erotic enough to generate increased levels of adrenalin and endorphins and provide the girl with the feeling of being submissive to her masterful lover—or vice versa. Roles can be reversed. She cracks the whip, and becomes the dominatrix.

Pain itself is a relative sensation. For some, even the lightest spanking would be unpleasant and definitely not erotic. Others may prefer a sharper sensation. Whether it's nails raking across sensitized flesh or teeth grazing a hardened nipple, or the feel of a leather as it warms an exposed buttock, what is "too much" pain is truly up to the receiver. Be sure to discuss this with your partner. Communication is key, to ensure the sensation doesn't go from erotic to unpleasant.

Bondage, Discipline, Sadism & Masochism (BDSM)

With BDSM we are entering the realms of extreme fantasy. If practiced between willing partners, with a healthy attitude toward the difference between right and wrong, and founded in absolute trust in each other, it can add a dimension of heightened erotic thrills, which would be difficult to match.

Imagine the woman spread-eagle across the bed, in an X formation. Her hands and feet secured to each corner of the bed by ties and handcuffs.

IMPORTANT: In case of emergencies or objections, the handcuffs, or any other securing devices, must be easily freed by her without help.

This where you can begin. The woman is totally vulnerable, and the man is in total control.

There are far too many variations on this theme of tying up and being tied up, pseudo-punishment routines and being in or out of control, for me to list here. However, even reading about the many aspects of BDSM can be arousing. Look at the success of *Fifty Shades of Grey* by E. L. James. The first of a triology became a global best seller, with no conventional marketing, just by word of mouth, because of its BDSM content.

If you're interested and would like to read a sensible approach to BDSM, I highly recommend Ten Tips for Bringing BDSM Into Your Bedroom, by the delightful author and romance writer Joey W Hill, as a good starting point. You'll find her narrative here: http://thecelebritycafe.com/feature/2012/09/ten-tips-bringing-bdsm-your—bedroom.

Body Alterations

For primarily the under-40 demographic, body alterations are a popular fetish. Piercings, tattoos and surgical implants can cause a thrum of desire in some. Tongue, nipple and genital piercings can not only be physically attractive to potential partners with this fetish, but also these piercings can come into play during times of intimacy, contributing to the popularity of this fetish. A fetish for body piercings and tattoos is known as stigmatophilia.

Tip: Avoid imitation tongue piercings. These are two, small decoratively produced pieces that contain very strong magnets. When positioned on either side of the tongue, the magnets hold them together, making them appear to be a piercing. They're not infallible. If dislodged and swallowed, they can become life-threatening, when they reach your intestines, by clamping sections of your intestines together and forming a blockage.

Sensual Materials

A fondness for leather attracts many men and women alike. Whether it's a woman clad in form-fitting leather pants or a man sporting a bad boy leather jacket, even the smell can cause arousal. Entire nightclubs are based on the leather fetish. Of course, there are other materials fetishes are based upon. Fur, latex, rubber, and silk— either worn or used to stroke a partner's skin—have numerous fetish fans. Marilyn Monroe, for example, would only sleep on silk sheets.

Shoes

For inanimate object fetishes, shoes are one of the most common—from strappy heels to over-the-knee boots. This is mostly a male fetish, and it primarily involves women wearing high heels, often during sex. The facets of the shoe's design is important to the shoe fetishist—the height of the heel, the pointiness of the toe, the length of the shaft of the boot. A fetish for high heels specifically is known as altocalciphilia.

Feet

Those with a foot fetish can be aroused by feet, toes or even shoes. In fact, some research indicate more people reported having a foot fetish than those with breast or butt fetishes.[136] Like leather clubs, there are entire clubs devoted to the foot fetishist. Also known as podophilia, foot fetishism, like shoes, is mostly a male fetish. The shape and size of the foot, foot jewelry (such as toe rings) and even the odor of the foot can be erotic to many. Licking and kissing the foot, sucking on toes, massaging, or even tickling can provide sexual pleasure to both parties with a foot fetish.

Voyeurism

Watching other people having sex, generally without their knowledge—voyeurism—is also known as scopophilia or scoptophilia. There's another form of voyeurism that involves watching oneself using mirrors.

I knew an Arab Prince who had a house not far from mine. He bought a Tudor period house and had it totally refurbished inside. The master bedroom had a ceiling crisscrossed with oak beams. Within the squares, created between those beams, he had mirrors fixed. As you entered the room the mirrors, hidden between the beams, were not apparent. However, as soon as you lay on his Prince-sized bed and looked at the ceiling, you were presented with reflected images of the entire bed. Whoever lay on their back missed nothing!

Balloons

Rolling around with inflated balloons, pressing them between bodies, sometimes bursting them is another fetish. Having a fetish about inanimate objects, especially with a pronounced emotional desire, is known as objectophilia.

Bad Language

Using foul or obscene words is known as narratophilia. Users of this fetish can become highly aroused by using bad language. It can work both ways as well. I had a lengthy interview with a well-spoken, educated woman and whilst quietly spoken, she unexpectedly used the word 'fucking' in conversation. I found this to be strangely arousing!

Feederism

Feederism centers on erotic eating and feeding involving placing edible substances, like cream or chocolate spreads, on erogenous body parts and having your partner eat or lick them off.

Enemas

Either giving or having an enema can be a turn on for some, and is known as klismaphilia.

Transvestism

Transvestism is the wearing of clothes associated with the opposite sex. Transvestophilia is the desire for a transvestite sexual partner.

Exhibitionism

Exhibitionism is where a person, of either sex, goes naked in front of others, often in a public place. Many will have witnessed a 'streaker' running across a soccer ground during a game. In front of a sporting crowd this is usually met with shouts of approval, or derision if interfering with the game's progress, but the place and timing are important if not to offend anyone.

Extremes

While traveling the Far East, I came across a club for deviant gentlemen. A popular pastime with some was to have a girl defecate onto a glass-topped table, while they lay underneath to watch. The girls were highly paid to eat only herbs for a week before performing this act—so no objectionable smells.

For another example of how a fetish can go to an extreme, come with me to the Black Museum at Scotland Yard. While visiting, the curator showed me various 'tools' used for practicing sadomasochism, including a police truncheon with a spiral of barbed wire wrapped around it.[137] Enough said.

Taking Fetish Too Far

Between two (or more) consenting adults, fetish and fantasy can create a diverse, exciting and fulfilling sex life. However, when a person inflicts their fetish or fantasy on others, without their permission, fetish can go too far . . . and even become illegal.

Danger and Excitement

Being placed in a position of danger—either deliberately or accidentally—can produce sexual arousal. You might discover this when being robbed or held up, in which case it is known as chremastistophilia.

Rubbing Against a Non-Consenting Person

This fetish, described as frotteurism, is most often read about in newspapers. It is illegal in most situations.

Penis Exposure

Even if you've never seen a "flasher," you likely know the stereotypical image. A man in a raincoat approaches you and opens his coat to reveal his naked body, complete with an erect penis. Exposing one's penis is called peodektophilia. Compared to other crimes, you may think this is a pretty harmless occurrence. However, in most places, exposing yourself to others in public is illegal. It can also be psychologically damaging to those who've been subjected to the exposure.

Of course, some handle a situation like this better than others. There was a secretary I knew working out of a London office who seemed to attract more than her fair share of flashers. Because it happened so often she developed a simple put-down. As the flasher exposed himself she exclaimed, "My, my, what a little one!" It worked every time.

Erotic Asphyxiation

Also known as auto-erotic asphyxiation, it is said being unable to breathe at the point of orgasm heightens the experience to levels unattainable by any other means. I am not about to corroborate this view. The methods used are far too dangerous in my view, and people die from this fetish. They usually achieve reaching the point of unconsciousness by covering their head with a plastic bag or strangulation, making breathing impossible. Death would only be seconds away.

DO NOT TRY THIS!

The point is, when taken too far fetishes can be psychologically, and sometimes physically, harmful to others, as well as yourself. No matter what your particular fetish, having full consent from your partner is critical. This goes beyond the initial agreement to take part in a particular fetish-based activity, and includes a continued consent throughout your session.

Consent

"Safe words"—words chosen before you begin, and indicates one person wants to stop immediately, no questions asked, are critical to ensure emotional and physical safety. You must always, always have respect for your partner(s) and be especially careful of the trust they put in you when they indulge your fetishes and fantasies.

In Summary

For most people it is the simplest things that can prompt sexual arousal. Just because they might be labeled 'a fetish' doesn't mean you're weird or perverted. It is totally natural. There are numerous tricks of the mind as well as physical aids—bodily or mechanical—that can get us in the mood or speed us on our way to a climax.

The smell of his cologne, her favorite perfume, the dimples in her cheeks, the way she walks, all of these things can be described as fetishes when you know they can trigger a sexual desire. Swimming in the nude can be an exhilarating experience; not everyone likes to but to some the feeling of the water flowing over their bodies, and over their genitals in particular, can produce a sexual desire. Yes, the clinical guys even have a name for this—but who cares when they get the urge!

The acceleration of 400 tonnes of a Boeing 747 thrusting me back into my seat at take-off still raises the hairs on the back of my neck; for some it may raise more than this. But as a kid it was the vibration of the school bus engine felt through the seat of my pants that sexually excited me, and I know of girls who admit to having the same experience.

If you know what excites you, you are fortunate. If you can tap into those very private resources, you are blessed. If you discover some external situations—from environment to toys—provide extra enjoyment, you are quite normal.

Don't let it worry you if what tickles you doesn't necessarily tickle your friends. But do talk about those things with your partner; you may discover new 'buttons' to press that get each other going.

—— 22 ——

Conception and Contraception

Familiarity breeds contempt—and children.

~ Mark Twain

It's easy to forget, when writing about sex, that nature's prime objective in getting two people of opposite genders to mate (copulate, fuck, etc.) is to procreate—to produce children and continue the species.

For generations, we have been fortunate to have the means to enjoy sex without causing pregnancy. This has allowed us to spend time examining and practicing what pleasures us and our partners most, while forgetting all about how or why we got there in the first place.

If no contraceptive precautions are taken, and the male sperm is allowed to take its intended journey, pregnancy can result. Earlier in this book, we discovered the mechanics of ejaculation, but what happens after that?

Dr Michael Mosley takes up the story:

As many as 250 million sperm start the journey into the woman's body, but very few will make it to the egg. Sperm are alien and the woman's immune system is triggered to kill them!

White blood cells attack the sperm from all directions. By the time any survivors reach the safety of a fallopian tube, from the original 250 million there could be as few as twenty left.

It might seem odd but it's an incredibly effective selection process. And it clearly works because humans can be extremely successful breeders.

All women have only a limited supply of eggs. A woman is born with all the eggs she will ever have. It's a strange thought, but the egg that started you, started life in your grandmother! It means that the egg that made you was inside your mother when she was just a fetus inside her mother.

The precious egg that made you was stored inside your mother's ovaries for decades. Then, when its time came, it rose to the surface and ripened.

As soon as an egg is ripe it's released from the ovary, and gently released into the opening of the fallopian tube. The sperm are now in a race to the finish. They have come a long way, but there can be only one winner. The competing sperm break off the cloud of cells that surround the egg. They struggle to find a way in—until one manages to break through the soft shell underneath. This is a critical moment for the egg. If a second sperm gets in, the egg won't survive. It must quickly protect itself. Under the shell tiny granules detonate, hardening it and making the egg impenetrable.

A new life is under way.[138]

Contraception

Early Methods

Contraception isn't a new idea. Preventing unwanted pregnancies have been a concern for generations. An early Aboriginal method of contraception pierced the underside of the penis at its root. They then plugged the pierced hole with a wooden plug. The plug was left in place so urinating remained normal. However, when erect and intending to make love, the plug was removed, which allowed the ejaculate to drain out from the hole in the base of the penis, instead of being deposited inside the woman's vagina. If the Aboriginal man wanted to impregnate his partner, the plug stayed in. Obviously this didn't prevent pregnancy 100 percent of the time, plus it was an incredibly painful procedure when the opening was created!

Male Condoms

Condoms have been used since the early days of the Roman Empire.[139] These first condoms were made from animal gut. Lambskin condoms (made from sheep intestine) are still used today, especially by people with latex allergies. However, lambskin condoms do NOT prevent viral STDs, like HIV or herpes.

Latex condoms, made from natural rubber latex, are the most common, due to the low cost and durability. There are also several brands now that offer synthetic latex, polyisoprene, to help those who have latex allergies. Polyurethane condoms are also available; however, they are typically very thin and can trigger an allergic reaction.

Male condoms are a thin sheath placed over an erect penis to keep sperm from entering a woman's body. Condoms work best when used with a vaginal spermicide, which kills any sperm that escape from the condom. Please note, you need to use a new condom with each sex act. NEVER re—use a condom.

Condoms come in a variety of sizes, and plethora of options. These include:

- Lubricated condoms,

- Non-lubricated,

PLEASE NOTE: *If you add lubrication to a non-lubricated condom, be sure to use a water-based lubricant, such as K-Y Jelly. Oil-based lubricants, including massage oils, baby oils, and petroleum jelly, can weaken the condom material and cause it to tear or break.*

- Flavored condoms for oral sex,

- Condoms in a variety of colors for the fashionable condom wearer (even glow-in-the dark!),

- Textured condoms with ribbing, bumps, and other textures "for her pleasure",

- Thicker condoms designed specifically for anal sex, and

- Even climax-control condoms with a desensitization cream that may be helpful for men who suffer from premature ejaculation.

Keep condoms in a cool, dry place. If you keep them in a hot place (like a wallet or glove compartment), the latex breaks down, and the condom can tear or break during use.

Withdrawal

One of the most obvious methods of contraception is the 'withdrawal' or 'pulling out' method. With this method, the penis is removed from the woman's vagina before ejaculation. The biggest challenge with this method is it takes a lot of self-control by the man. Also, as we know, sperm have a habit of creeping out of the penis, even before ejaculation, riding in the moisture that precedes ejaculation. Although withdrawal isn't completely reliable, it is still practiced by many, often due to unplanned opportunity.

The Rhythm Method

The rhythm method is a popular form of contraception for those who, for religious reasons, do not believe in the use of other forms of contraception. The rhythm method centers on a woman's menstrual cycle. By tracking changes in the woman's body, including dates of menstruation, body temperature and vaginal discharge, a woman may be able to predict which days of the month she is most fertile. By not having sex on these days, she is less likely to become pregnant. However, this method is usually only effective for women who have regular menstrual cycles, and even then is only 75 to 87 percent effective.[140] Also, the rhythm method does NOT protect against any sexually transmitted diseases.

Surgical Methods of Contraception

For men, the most common surgical method of contraception is the vasectomy. The vasectomy is considered a permanent form of birth control, although it can, in some instances, be surgically-reversed. The vas deferens is surgically cut, clamped or otherwise sealed, which prevents sperm from mixing with the semen. Without sperm in the semen, eggs cannot be fertilized. It may take several months for all of the remaining sperm to be ejaculated, so a second form of contraception is needed, shortly after the vasectomy, until a zero sperm count is achieved.

For women, tubal ligation (having your 'tubes tied') is the most common permanent, surgical method of contraception. In this procedure, the fallopian tubes, which carry the egg from the ovaries to the uterus, are tied, cut or blocked.

A new, non-surgical method works along the same theory of blocking the fallopian tube, with a tubal implant. These are small, metal coils that are inserted into the fallopian tubes. Scar tissue develops around the implant, usually within three months, and eventually permanently blocks the tube. A second form of birth control is needed until it is confirmed by x-ray the fallopian tubes are completely blocked.

Hormonal Methods of Contraception

Hormonal methods of contraception are very effective means of birth control and work by preventing the egg's release from the ovaries. This changes the lining in the uterus, so an egg cannot implant and changes the cervical mucus to form a barrier against sperm entering the uterus. There are two basic formulas for hormonal contraception:

- **Combination hormonal contraception, with both estrogen and progestin**—These include pills like 'The Pill,' skin patches, rings, and implants.

- **Progestin-only hormonal contraception**—These include mini—pills, shots such as the Depo shot, implants, and progestin-only IUD.

Combination pills taken for hormonal contraception are typically taken daily. Your doctor may advise you not to take the pill if you:

- Are older than 35 and smoke,

- Have a history of blood clots,

- Have a history of breast, liver, or endometrial cancer

Antibiotics may reduce how well the pill works in some women. Talk to your doctor about a backup method of birth control if you need to take antibiotics.

Women should wait three weeks after giving birth to begin using birth control that contains both estrogen and progestin. These methods increase the risk of dangerous blood clots, which could form after giving birth. Women who delivered by caesarean section or have other risk factors for blood clots, such as obesity, history of blood clots, smoking, or preeclampsia, should wait six weeks.

Rings, like the Nuva-Ring, allow a combination hormonal method of contraception, which you don't have to worry about daily. You squeeze the ring between your thumb and index finger and insert it into your vagina. You wear the ring for 3 weeks, take it out for the week that you have your period and then put in a new ring.

Implants are a matchstick-size, flexible rod put under the skin of the upper arm. It is often called by its brand name, Implanon. Implants are effective for up to 3 years.

Progestin-only shots, like the Depo shot, are given once every three months. The shot should not be used for more than two years in a row, because it can cause a temporary loss of bone density. The loss increases the longer this method is used. Bone does start to reform after this method is stopped; however, it may increase the risk of fracture and osteoporosis, if used for a long time.

An IUD is a small device shaped like a "T" that goes in your uterus. There are two types of IUDs:

- **Copper IUD**—The copper IUD goes by the brand name ParaGard.

  It releases a small amount of copper into the uterus, which prevents the sperm from reaching and fertilizing the egg. If fertilization does occur, the IUD keeps the fertilized egg from implanting in the lining of the uterus. A doctor needs to put in your copper IUD. It can stay in your uterus for 5 to 10 years.

- **Hormonal IUD**—The hormonal IUD goes by the brand name Mirena. It is sometimes called an intrauterine system, or IUS. It releases progestin into the uterus, which keeps the ovaries from releasing an egg and causes the cervical mucus to thicken so sperm can't reach the egg. It also affects the ability of a fertilized egg to successfully implant in the uterus. A doctor needs to put in a hormonal IUD. It can stay in the uterus for up to 5 years.

Barrier Methods for Women

In addition to men wearing a condom, there are barrier methods of contraception designed for women. These prevent the sperm from entering the uterus and reaching the egg. Although they are not as effective as hormonal methods of contraception, they do have fewer side effects. By adding spermicides and condoms, the effectiveness of female barrier methods can be increased. Female barrier methods include:

- **Diaphragm**—a shallow, latex cup that prevents sperm from traveling to the uterus,

- **Cervical Cap**—a thimble-shaped latex cup. It is often called by its brand name, FemCap,

- **Cervical Shield**—a silicone cup that has a one-way valve that creates suction and helps it fit against the cervix. It is often called by its brand name, Lea's Shield,

- **Female Condoms**—This condom is worn by the woman inside her vagina. It keeps sperm from getting into her body. It is made of thin, flexible manmade rubber and is packaged with a lubricant. It can be inserted up to 8 hours before having sex. Use a new condom each time you have intercourse. And don't use it and a male condom at the same time,

- **Spermicidal Gel or Foam**—most often nonoxynol-9, which kills sperm, is inserted into the vaginal canal to kill any sperm that enter the vagina, and

- **Sponge**—This barrier method is a soft, disk-shaped device with a loop for taking it out. It is made out of polyurethane foam and contains the spermicide nonoxynol-9. Spermicide kills sperm. Before having sex, you wet the sponge and place it, loop side down, inside your vagina to cover the cervix. The sponge is effective for more than one act of intercourse, for up to 24 hours. It needs to be left in for at least 6 hours after having sex to prevent pregnancy. The sponge must then be taken out within 30 hours after it is inserted.

The diaphragm and cervical cap come in different sizes, and you need a doctor to "fit" you for one. The cervical shield and sponges come in one size, and you will not need a fitting.

Things to Consider

Before choosing a birth control method, think about:

- Your overall health

- How often you have sex

- The number of sex partners you have

- If you want to have children someday

- How well each method works to prevent pregnancy

- Possible side effects

- Your comfort level with using the method

Keep in mind, even the most effective birth control methods can fail. However, your chances of getting pregnant are lowest if the method you choose is always used correctly and every time you have sex.

No matter what method you use, it is important to remember the only guaranteed way to avoid STIs (Sexually transmitted Infections), STDs (Sexually Transmitted Diseases), or what used to be referred to as VD (Venereal Disease), is total abstinence. Of course, if you've picked up this book, chances are abstinence is not your lifestyle of choice.

Apart from total abstinence, the only safe way to avoid STDs is to always use a condom. Even with a condom, you have to remember the vagina is not the only orifice that can receive or transmit STDs. Your mouth and anus are also prime places of infection. In fact, actor Michael Douglas' has stated his throat cancer was directly due to oral sex. For this reason, until you settle down with a monogamous life-partner, always consider the disease prevention as well as pregnancy prevention, when selecting a form of birth control.

More Information

More information on birth control methods (in the U.S.) can be obtained by visiting www.womenshealth.gov or calling them at 800-994-9662 (TDD: 888-220-5446) or contact the following organizations:

American College of Obstetricians and Gynecologists

Phone: 800-762-2264 x 349 (for publications requests only)

Food and Drug Administration—www.fda.gov

Phone: 888-463-6332

Planned Parenthood Federation of America—www. plannedparenthood.org/

Phone: 800-230-7526

Population Council—www.popcouncil.org/

Phone: 212-339-0500

—— 23 ——

Problem Solving

*No problem can be solved from the same level
of consciousness that created it.*

~ Albert Einstein

Imbalance of Desire

We all go through anxious periods, when sex disappears off the list of life's priorities. Sometimes this happens with both partners. At other times, this only happens for one. Imbalance in desire between partners can cause friction at best, divorce at worst.

The answer here is to talk to each other. If you're always on the defensive, this can lead to coldness and withdrawal. The next time you're chatting about personal things, to help prevent your partner from going on the defensive, say, "I feel . . ." not "You make me feel." If you're having difficulty in finding the time or ways of introducing intimate subjects into conversation, you might find the answer in the chapter on Communication.

There could be one or more of a hundred reasons why one partner just doesn't want to have sex with you as frequently, or even at all, as you would like. There might be a simple answer. Talking about your perceived problem openly and honestly should bring about at least an understanding and quite often a solution.

This isn't to say you and your partner must match libidos exactly. For most, this ideal is as distant as the moon. However, understanding the imbalance and applying love and compassion can provide the answer. As an example, if you are a woman and enjoy coupling with your partner once a week, but he would prefer three times a week, suggest you provide release for him without actually having intercourse. You don't even have to take your clothes off; you can fellate him or masturbate him a couple of times a week and still enjoy full passionate sex with him on the regular basis you prefer. The same reasoning applies if the gender preferences are reversed. Such practices have been known to increase desire for more frequent sex by those administering the interim quickies.

Winter Blues[141]

Problem One: Hibernation Instinct

You are biologically programmed to lose your sex drive in winter. You can thank your ancestors' hibernation patterns for your winter libido drop, a University of Tasmania study found. "Hibernation caused their metabolisms to slow and sex drives to wane, as they increased their calorie load and slept more," says the study's co-author Dr Margaret Austen. Thanks a lot, Darwinism.

Seasonal Affective Disorder (SAD): The Solution

Trick your body into thinking it's still summer by investing in a blue-light light bulb. While splashing out on a pricey light-therapy box used to be one way of getting her in a better mood, and thus *in* the mood, studies reported in the *Journal of Clinical Endocrinology and Metabolism* have found a simple blue light is twice as effective.

Blue light resets the body's circadian rhythms by tricking it into thinking it's a bright summer's day. You can purchase blue lights from a variety of online light therapy retailers, including http://www.sad.co.uk. If you don't want to give your room an icy glow, download the BluWave application to your iPhone or BlueLight for your Droid phone.

What Not to Do

If you suffer from SAD, don't try to cheer yourself up with a drink. Studies published in the *American Journal of Physiology* have found drinking alcohol affects your body's "master clock" and disrupts your energy levels further, making the problem worse—not better.

Problem Two: Cold Weather

Cold weather dulls sexual sensations. Lower body temperatures dampen arousal for both men and women. "If your skin is warmer, it's more sensitive," says Dr. Ian Kerner, sexual therapist and author of *She Comes First*. "Most men will notice that when they get cold, their penis will shrink," says Kerner. See, you're not the only one!

The Solution

It's a great excuse to take someone else's clothes off. Nothing heats you up faster than someone else's body heat, according to University of Illinois studies. "Plus, skin-to skin contact boosts the levels of oxytocin—women's feel-good hormone, so acts as an aphrodisiac," says Kerner. Bonus points: nude sleeping means no struggling with her bra clasp.

What Not to Do

Don't forget to tell her to keep her socks on. Women are 30% more likely to orgasm if they keep their feet warm, discovered Dutch scientists from the University of Groningen.

Problem Three: Christmas Dinner

Winter weight gain zaps your sex drive. There's a biological reason why your summer six-pack is buried under winter's spare tire. Studies by Indiana University have found that men pile on a minimum of at least 2 pounds or 1 kilogram over the winter because cold weather makes you want to eat more. Unfortunately for you, a study by Duke University showed gaining weight kills libido and makes both men and women less sexually adventurous.

The Solution

Boost your levels of sex and happiness hormones with a meat-feast pizza. You don't have to ditch the filling winter fare—just eat smarter. Studies published in *The Lancet* have shown that levels of serotonin are lowest in the winter and highest on bright, sunny days. However, according to University of North Carolina studies, it is possible to replicate the summer serotonin boost by watching what you eat. The scientists found that serotonin is manufactured from protein-rich foods and its release is triggered by carbohydrates. That smells to us like a meat-feast pizza!

Don't forget the Chianti. Scientists from the University of Florence reported women who drank wine with their meals had higher sex drives and reported stronger orgasms.

What Not to Do

Don't try to give her libido a boost by loading up on dessert. Scientists from St. Vincent's University Hospital in Dublin found that in reality eating a sugary snack can temporarily lower your testosterone levels, which in turn can zap your sex drive, whether male or female. Even chocolate, that rumored aphrodisiac, isn't all its mythical status purports.

Although chocolate has two chemicals ascribed to aphrodisiac qualities—tryptophan and phenlethylamine, there are insufficient quantities of these substances in chocolate to have any measurable effect on desire. Studies have yet to link chocolate and desire, in fact, one Italian study of 163 women found no differences in desire between women who consumed three or more servings of chocolate per day and those who only consumed one serving per day[142].

Distractions

Television

It's not surprising that experts believe a television in the bedroom is bad for your sex life. Many people, men included, can be put off their stroke by a distraction at the wrong moment.

As I've said before, the best sex is achieved when your mind, especially hers, is completely devoid of any mundane thoughts—apart from sexual ones, of course—and uninterrupted peace and quiet is required. If you must have a live screen in the room, put on some erotic or pornographic (if you are both in agreement on this) images on to help build your journey. Otherwise, switch it off.

Turn-Offs

Apart from the visual and audible interruptions, attention to other possible distractions is also worthwhile. Having to scramble around looking for lubricating gel or a condom still in its wrapper can spoil the moment. Organize before you get started. If the kids are about, lock the bedroom door.

Hygiene

Napoleon was famously quoted as sending a message to Josephine, saying he was returning home and requested she not wash for three days before he arrived. Although I can understand a man finding his lover's body perfume erotic, I very much doubt three days without washing would be found attractive by any man—especially in those bygone days of poor sanitation; forgive me if you are the exception.

Ignore nothing when bathing. Showering can be most effective but still wash and rinse, at least twice, the genitalia and anal areas. Squat to open up those places where fingers and tongues might explore and wash again. Under arms can be troublesome; wash and check them out.

While careful attention is required around the vulva, washing *inside* the vagina is not necessary or good for you. The vagina is self—cleaning and lubricating and should be left that way. Fluids produced in the vagina are also part of the body's defense mechanism against fungal, bacterial, and viral invaders; not to be washed away.

Unless you're under the shower together, drying is as important as washing. Spread your thighs and towel thoroughly. Blow-dry with legs spread, especially if hairy down there. Dampness, unless produced by natural love juices through joint sexual exertion, can be a turn-off for some, and a warm, damp hairy place is a perfect home for bacteria—and those little devils work really fast at producing bad odors.

Oral Hygiene

Don't forget your mouth is a big reservoir of bacteria. Mind what you eat. Spicy food will encourage smelly breath. Garlic and onions are also culprits of lingering mouth odor.

It has been said kissing a smoker is like kissing an ashtray. Don't smoke—it not only stinks and leaves your hair, skin and clothes smelling but is also very bad for your overall health and sexual health. It narrows the arteries. Poor blood flow causes loss of erection in men and loss of sensitivity in women, in addition to being carcinogenic—AKA cancer causing.

Keep your mouth clean, use a mouthwash and brush and floss your teeth at least twice a day, preferably after eating.

Cystitis

Cystitis is a urinary tract infection causing inflammation of the bladder. The most common symptom is a burning feeling when you're urinating. Another symptom is the need to pee often. If left untreated, the symptoms get worse.

The cause of cystitis is an infection on the skin surface around the opening of the urinary tract, which is about 2 inches (52mm) long in women and about 8 inches (210mm) in men. The shorter urinary tract is the reason for women suffering more readily from this problem than men.

Although easily cured—see your doctor or pharmacist as soon as you suspect an infection and they will supply antibiotic treatment and it will clear up within 4 to 9 days—avoidance is better. That's why I've written about the importance of oral hygiene. The transfer of bacteria from mouth to urinary tract can occur during cunnilingus (giving head) or fellatio (blow job)!

Bladder Issues: What You need to know about Bladder Control for Women[143]

Women of all ages have bladder control problems.

Urine Leakage: A Common Health Problem for Women of All Ages

You may think bladder control problems are something that happens only when you get older. The truth is women of all ages have urine leakage. The problem is also called incontinence. Men leak urine too, but the problem is more common in women.

- Many women leak urine when they exercise, laugh hard, cough, or sneeze, (and during sexual intercourse).

- Often women leak urine when they are pregnant or after they have given birth.

- Women who have stopped having their periods— menopause—often report bladder control problems.

- Female athletes of all ages sometimes have urine leakage during strenuous sports activities. [including approaching orgasm]

Urine leakage may be a small bother or a large problem. About half of adult women say they have had urine leakage at one time or another. Many women say it's a daily problem.

Urine leakage is more common in older women, but that doesn't mean it's a natural part of aging. You don't have to "just live with it." You can do something about it and regain your bladder control.

Incontinence is not a disease. But it may be a sign that something is wrong. It's a medical problem, and a doctor or nurse can help.

How Does the Bladder Work?

The bladder is a balloon-shaped organ that stores and releases urine. It sits in the pelvis. The bladder is supported and held in place by pelvic muscles. The bladder itself is a muscle.

Parts of the Bladder Control System

The tube that carries urine from your body is called the urethra. Ring-like muscles called sphincters help keep the urethra closed so urine doesn't leak from the bladder before you're ready to release it.

Several body systems must work together to control the bladder.

1. Pelvic floor muscles hold the bladder in place.

2. Sphincter muscles keep the urethra closed.

3. The bladder muscle relaxes when it fills with urine and squeezes when it's time to urinate. the bladder is full.

4. Nerves carry signals from the bladder to let the brain know when the bladder is full.

5. Nerves also carry signals from the brain to tell the bladder when it's time to urinate.

6. Hormones help keep the lining of the bladder and urethra healthy.

Figure 19: Side and Bottom View of Female Pelvic Region

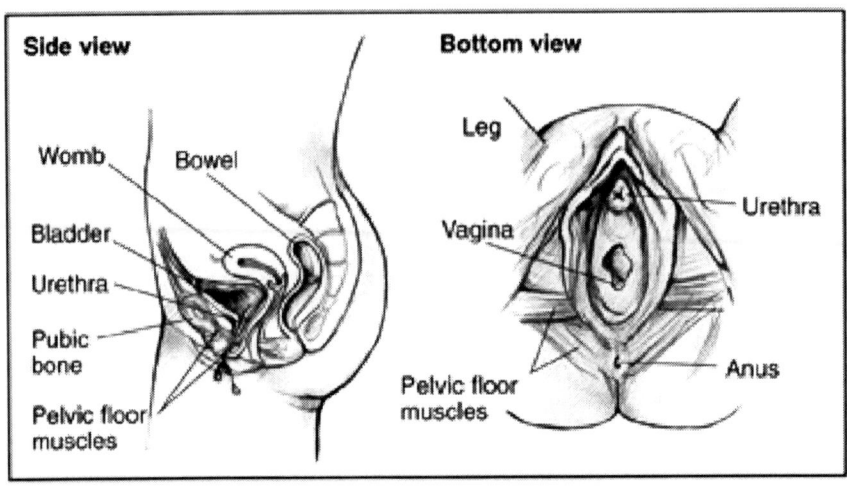

Bladder control problems can start when any one of these features is not working properly.

Parts of the Bladder Control System: Nerves and Brain

What are the different types of bladder control problems?

Not all bladder control problems are alike. Some problems are caused by weak muscles, while others are caused by damaged nerves. Sometimes the cause may be a medicine that dulls the nerves.

To help solve your problem, your doctor or nurse will try to identify the type of incontinence you have. It may be one or more of the following six types:

- **Temporary Incontinence**—As the name suggests, temporary incontinence doesn't last. You may have an illness, like a urinary tract infection, that causes frequent and sudden urination that you can't control. Or you may find that a new medicine has the unexpected side effect of increasing your urination. These problems go away as soon as the cause is found and corrected.

- **Stress Incontinence**—If you leak urine when you cough, laugh, sneeze, or exercise, you have stress incontinence. Mental stress does not cause stress incontinence. The "stress" is pressure on the bladder. When your pelvic and sphincter muscles are strong, they can handle the extra pressure from a cough, sneeze, exercise, or laugh. But when those muscles are weak, that sudden pressure can push urine out of the bladder. In stress incontinence, weak pelvic muscles can let urine escape when a cough or other action puts pressure on the bladder.

- **Urge Incontinence**—If you leak urine after a strong, sudden urge to urinate, you have urge incontinence. This bladder control problem may be caused by nerve damage from diabetes, a stroke, an infection, or another medical condition.

- **Mixed Incontinence**—Mixed incontinence is a mix of stress and urge incontinence. You may leak urine with a laugh or sneeze at one time. At another time you may have a sudden, uncontrollable urge to urinate just before you leak.

- **Functional Incontinence**—Some people have trouble getting to the bathroom. If you have urine leakage because you can't walk or have other mobility problems, you have functional incontinence.

- **Overactive Bladder**—If you have to urinate eight or more times a day, you may have an overactive bladder. Getting up to urinate two or more times each night is another sign of overactive bladder. With an overactive bladder, you feel strong, sudden urges to urinate, and you may also have urge incontinence.

What Causes Bladder Control Problems?

Urine leakage has many possible causes. However, most bladder control problems are caused by weak pelvic muscles. These muscles may become stretched and weak during pregnancy and childbirth. Weak muscles let the bladder sag out of position, which may stretch the opening to the urethra.

Damaged nerves may also send signals to the bladder at the wrong time. As a result, a bladder spasm may push out urine without warning. Sometimes damaged nerves send no signals at all, and the brain can't tell when the bladder is full. Nerves can be damaged by disease or trauma.

Diseases and conditions that can damage the nerves include:

1. Diabetes

2. Parkinson's

3. Multiple sclerosis

4. Stroke

Trauma that can damage the nerves include:

1. Pelvic or back surgery

2. Herniated disc

3. Radiation

4. Medicines, alcohol, and caffeine. Leaking can happen when medicines affect any of the muscles or nerves. You may take medicine to calm your nerves so that you can sleep or relax. This medicine may dull the nerves in the bladder and keep them from signalling the brain when the bladder is full. Without the message and urge, the bladder overflows. Drinking alcohol can also cause these nerves to fail. Water, pills, diuretics, take fluid from the swollen areas of your body and send it to the bladder. This rapid filling may cause the bladder to leak. Caffeine drinks such as coffee and cola also cause the bladder to fill quickly. Make sure your drinks are decaf.

5. Infection. A urinary tract infection can irritate bladder nerves and cause the bladder to squeeze without warning. This type of incontinence goes away once the infection has been cured.

6. Excess weight. Being overweight can put pressure on the bladder and contribute to stress incontinence.

How Do I Tell My Health Care Team About My Urine Leakage?

Talking about bladder control problems is not easy for some people. You may feel embarrassed to tell your doctor. But talking about the problem is the first step in finding an answer. Also, you can be sure your doctor has heard it all before. You will not shock or embarrass your doctor or nurse.

Medical History

You can prepare for your visit to the doctor's office by gathering the information your doctor will need to understand your problem. Make a list of the medicines you are taking. Include prescription medicines and those you buy over the counter, like aspirin or antacid. List the fluids you drink regularly, including sodas, coffee, tea, and alcohol. Tell the doctor how much of each drink you have in an average day.

Finding a Doctor

You will need to find a doctor who is skilled in helping women with urine leakage. If your primary doctor shrugs off your problem with normal aging. For example, ask for a referral to a specialist—a urogynecologist or a urologist who specializes in treating female urinary problems. You may need to be persistent, or you may need to look to organizations to help to locate a doctor in your area.

Make a note of any recent surgeries or illnesses you have had. Let the doctor know how many children you have had. These events may or may not be related to your bladder control problem.

Finally, keep track of the times when you have urine leakage. Note what you were doing at the time. Were you coughing, laughing, sneezing, or exercising? Did you have an uncontrollable urge to urinate when you heard running water?

Physical Exam

The doctor will give you a physical exam to look for any health issues that may be causing your bladder control problem. Checking your reflexes can show possible nerve damage. You will give a urine sample so the doctor can check for a urinary tract infection. For women, the exam may include a pelvic exam. Tests may also include taking an ultrasound picture of your bladder. Or the doctor may examine the inside of your bladder using a cystoscope, a long thin tube that slides up into the bladder through the urethra.

Bladder Function Tests

Your exam may include one or more tests that involve filling the bladder with warm fluid to measure the pressure at which leakage may occur. One simple test is called a stress test. You simply relax and then cough strongly to see if urine escapes.

Any medical test can be uncomfortable. Bladder testing may sound embarrassing, but the health professionals who perform the tests will try to make you feel comfortable and give you as much privacy as possible.

How is Loss of Bladder Control Treated?

Your doctor will likely offer several treatment choices. Some treatments are as simple as changing some daily habits. Other treatments require taking medicine or using a device. If nothing else seems to work, surgery may help a woman with stress incontinence regain her bladder control.

Talk with your doctor about which treatments might work best for you.

Pelvic Muscle Strengthening

Many women prefer to try the simplest treatment choices first. Kegel exercises strengthen the pelvic muscles and don't require any equipment. Once you learn how to "Kegel," you can Kegel anywhere. The trick is finding the right muscles to squeeze. Your doctor or nurse can help make sure you are squeezing the right muscles. Your doctor may refer you to a specially trained physical therapist who will teach you to find and strengthen the sphincter muscles. Learning when to squeeze these muscles can also help stop the bladder spasms that cause urge incontinence. After about 6 to 8 weeks, you should notice that you have fewer leaks and more bladder control. (Also read the chapter "Love Muscle")

You can do Kegel exercises while lying down, sitting at a desk, or standing up.

Erectile Dysfunction (ED)

There are many causes for a poor, or even non-existent, erection. It's frustrating for both partners but particularly depressing—even frightening—for the man. Compassionate understanding by the woman, and encouragement to discuss the problem with a medical practitioner, is essential. What is not helpful is a doubting woman who thinks it is because her partner no longer loves her; she is not attractive enough to get him excited; or has doubts about her 'expertise' in the bedroom. None of this is going to be true—I promise!

Go to the chapter on "The Penis" for explanations and steps to take to effect a remedy.

Peyronie's Disease

This doesn't affect every man, but the numbers it does affect warrant giving it a mention. Peyronie's describes a penis that has an unusual curve or bend making it uncomfortable, even painful, when erect and certainly difficult or impossible to use in penetrative sex.

The causes of this distressing disease are debatable—from a trauma to the penis, like accidentally bending it sharply during sexual activity or being hit in a car accident to a bodily malfunction that produces a fibrous thickening of tissue at a specific point which acts like scar tissue pulling at either end of the tissue and making the penis bend at that point.

A good example of a parallel disease that usually affects the hands of sufferers is Dupuytren's Disease—the thickening of fibrous tissue connecting fingers to the palm of the hand. This causes the fingers to claw down toward the palm—making it impossible to straighten out the affected finger(s). This is a similar effect as Peyronie's Disease in the penis.

Cures to straighten out the penis are varied and, once again, debatable. It depends on both the patient and the doctor as to which path they decide to take. For some, the answer is to simply wait and see, because Peyronie's has been known to correct itself. The body produces enzymes that reduce the fibrous tissue to an acceptable level and the penis becomes straighter and fully functional once again.

Surgery is a common treatment, where the offending tissue is simply removed and replaced with tissue harvested from another part of the patient's body. However, there is the risk of forming scar tissue which just brings the problem back again.

There is an alternative treatment using the manual exercise known as 'jelqing,' used by the penis enlargement fraternity as a method of increasing penis size. This method, used under the supervision of a physiotherapist, could be the answer for some.

Relationships

As we get older, and maybe too familiar and comfortable with our partner, it is just too easy to fall into routines that become habitual and acceptable. We forget, or even don't notice, what is fine and dandy with one may be lacking in excitement for the other.

It is all too easy to fall into a habit—quite unintentionally—of abstinence, maybe started by one partner suffering from a bad back or hacking cough. He or she sleeps in the spare bedroom, so the other partner can get a good night's sleep. In the worst scenarios, this becomes not just one night but many nights or even weeks, until the comfort of sleeping alone becomes the 'norm'.

Dr Gary Stollman Ph.D, a psychotherapist and author of _Relationship Stalemate: From Roommate to Soulmate_ was invited to comment on the film _Hope Springs_, starring Meryl Streep, Tommy Lee Jones and Steve Carell. He observed,

> _Sex becomes more routine, and advances to a stage when you begin to feel more like roommates. This can even get to a numbing relationship where you are just living out this routine._
>
> _This happens a lot—because many don't know how to keep a relationship alive._
>
> _Women tend to request help; men tend to shutdown, concentrate on work, keep busy; women communicate what they're feeling, unhappy, depressed, not feeling connected (so_

important)—and say they can't continue to live this way—and seek help from counseling experts.

The unique thing about therapy is that it is a safe environment—where couples can begin to talk about the real issues; therapy environment, and the security it provides, allows discussion of issues that have been put under the carpet. Until this, couples tend to shut themselves off not only from themselves but each other.

It's important to tell the person that they hurt you at the time that they hurt you. Or if something affects you, at the time that it affects you.

Don't hold it back; the longer you hold back the longer you become strangers to one another. When you can disclose those issues in a safe environment you can then move on past those issues and have a more vital relationship.

Sensate Sexercises (more information following this section) were created by Masters and Johnson many years ago. Sensate Focus is a way to reconnect with your partner by holding them, by touching them sensually but not sexually. These are steps couples have to move through to feel comfortable with one another and get used to being close again before moving into the sexual arena. It's very common, and very effective.

In every relationship there's always two "Is" and a "We". There has to be a balance between the "I" and the "We". Bring the "I" to the "We" and enrich that relationship much more. Do something new, different. If one can do this within a relationship for their partner, it can make all the difference in the world. Relationship is a process; if both are committed to make it work—to go that extra mile—if there's that little ounce of love underneath all that numbness that they feel—and they're willing to nurture—then they can get back to that place where they can experience that intimacy that they feel they have lost.[144]

Dr Stollman summarized the key elements to a successful relationship like this:

- To be true to our feelings.

- To express our feelings at the time that it happens.

- Add spice and romance to the relationship.

- Don't settle for less.

- If you want to make changes in your relationship you have to respect yourself.'

What 'intimacy' Dr Stollman refers to is, in my view, the superglue that holds us together. You see examples of this all around you; the strangest relationships that go beyond comprehension are always held together by the greatest intimacy.

Sensate Sexercises

Depending on where you live, and your circumstances, you can either seek a personal counselor or seek help from organizations like 'Relate' (www.relate-institute.org). You begin online by filling out their questionnaire. You might initially discuss your situation with your medical practitioner and ask for a referral to a counselor. Whatever route you decide to take, do it together. One-sided partnerships don't work. Looking into the matter subjectively and together does work.

However, if you and your partner feel your bedroom pleasures are completely off—and you have even reached a stage where you can't be bothered to try anymore—perhaps the subject is too embarrassing to discuss, because it has been so long. There is a glimmer of hope though, because you are reading this page!

Sit down with each other, follow the tips given so far and talk it over. Choose a time and place that both of you agree to ahead of time. Make a promise this first approach to what might have become a 'forgotten' subject will not lead to any attempt at sexual intercourse of any kind at that time. It is important that you do agree that the ideas discussed are aimed at getting your old intimacy back on track.

For the curious, here are a couple of examples of sexercises employed to suitable partnerships. Please note, each couple must have a program designed specifically for them—we are all different and have differing needs!

Sexercise Programs

Having got over the first hurdle, here are a couple of things you can try—at no cost and in the privacy of your own bedroom. You may be sleeping in separate beds or even separate rooms—for these sexercises you must at least be in the same room and, preferably, sharing a bed. If this is not possible, the sexercises can still be carried out, perhaps on a comfortable floor, but in a room with complete privacy and absolutely no interruptions. Turn off the radio/tv/phone.

Select a time that is not your usual bed-time. You'll choose an afternoon or evening with 30 minutes devoted each day for five days—all without sexual intercourse. There can be no breaks in this routine; keep disciplined.

- **Day One:** Lie next to each other, fully clothed, hand—touching or holding only and without talking. Just relax.

- **Day Two:** Lie next to each other, fully clothed, and gently caress each other's shoulders and arms for fifteen minutes, then kiss and cuddle for the remaining 15 minutes in the spooning position. No touching any erogenous areas—just relax and take it easy.

- **Day Three:** Undress, but keep your underwear on. Lie next to each other for the first 10 minutes holding hands only. Then begin gentle caresses of each others' arms and legs, starting at the shoulders and running down the arms and, with the legs, starting at the knees and running down to the feet. Taking it in turns avoids getting tangled in each other's limbs. Include some soft caressing of necks and running fingers through hair and conclude in the spooning position.

- **Day Four:** This is your first day of lying together totally naked. You are not to touch genitalia or breasts. Just softly caressing hair and heads, shoulders and arms, legs (no higher than the knees) and feet. Stop when you both agree to simply relax in the spooning position. Rest and relax a little, then begin caressing again until the 30 minutes is up.

- **Day Five:** Naked again, take the soft caresses over the erogenous areas. Do not go beyond any boundaries set by your partner. Do not involve any penetration. Do tease with your hands; pay particular attention to backs, buttocks, inner thighs, back of the knees ankles and feet. Gently kiss any part of the body, but avoid breasts and genitals. If either of you have feelings of arousal, that's a sign your libido is rising, but today you will remain celibate. Relax and look into each others' eyes frequently during this session.

- **Day Six:** Don't *plan* to have sex—intercourse is a natural thing, so just let it happen. Don't fight it, and don't force it. When it happens, it may be wonderful, or it may be mediocre. Don't worry about messing up—it happens all the time to all of us. It's only negative if you allow your mind to be negative.

. . . . On The Next Day

Do not jump on each other and have intercourse the moment you climb into the bed. Today you take the sharing of sensuality a stage further; employ all the moves of foreplay but never rush it.

Whisper in each others' ears about your sensual feelings; tell each other how good it feels to be so close. Look into each other's eyes, and see if you both agree to move on to full sex. Don't press the moment. Savor it and agree to go the full coupling the next day if uncertain.

Finally wrap yourselves in each others' arms—side-by-side is good, especially if you have a significant weight difference—and kiss and cuddle.

But do not rush it! Take your time. Listen to each other's breathing. Disappointment is easily achieved through anxiety. Be caring. Above all, be loving, and have fun. Too many people nowadays have forgotten how fun sex can be—smiling, laughing, being awkward, getting it wrong, feeling ecstasy—it's all part of sex. Enjoy it!

If you can't agree to full sex by now, you really should seek counseling.

Lovers Steeple

With both you and your partner naked, sit with legs crossed, on the floor or (firm) bed, facing each other, as close as you can get. I realize not many of us can take up the actual lotus position. However, tuck your feet up close to your thighs, in as comfortable position as you can, so your hands are free.

Raise both hands to shoulder level and, spreading your fingers out, touch finger tips only—thus making the form of a church steeple. Now look into each other's left eye, and hold that stare without speaking, for 5 minutes. The left eye thing is not as weird as you may think—try it and you will discover why. You don't have to be in need of any help or counseling to enjoy this exercise. It's especially good for those who like getting into their partner's mind, and it's a good way to relax after a hard day at work or with the children.

Female Sexual Dysfunction

This subject has, and continues to be, much debated. As you might expect, having achieved such success in recent years with drugs for men to overcome erectile dysfunction, the pharmaceutical industry has been working hard to find a drug that would heighten women's desire for sex.

As I've said before, drugs that dilate blood vessels feeding the penis in men, thus producing an erection, will also dilate the blood vessels of women in the pelvic region. However, the big difference is, although effective in aiding a man's desire for sex, it does nothing to increase desire in women.

It is a woman's mind that affects her desire—aided by an active libido.

Libido

Unlocking the mysteries of the female libido (and by so doing helping those women who suffer from lack of sexual desire) has been the subject of studies by many scientists. One such is Dr. Barry Komisaruk, a neuroscientist based at Rutgers University in New Jersey. Dr. Komisaruk heads up a research team that hopes to use their findings to pinpoint what is going wrong in those suffering sexual dysfunction or low libido.

As part of his research program, eight women were asked to stimulate themselves while lying under a blanket inside an MRI scanner. Monitoring the scanners images to see which parts became active, they discovered that sexual stimulus affects up to thirty different parts of the brain, including those responsible for emotion, touch, joy, satisfaction, and memory.

The research showed two minutes before orgasm, the brain's reward centers became active—these are the areas usually activated when eating food and drink. Immediately before orgasm, other areas of the brain became affected. These included: the sensory cortex, which receives 'touch' messages from parts of the body, and the thalamus, which relays signals to other parts of the body.

During orgasm, different parts of the brain were activated. These included those areas responsible for emotion. The final part to be activated was the hypothalamus, the 'control' part of the brain, which regulates temperature, hunger, thirst, and tiredness. At the same time, two more areas responsible for pleasure were activated plus another responsible for memory.

This research found the pattern of activity was the same for all women who participated in the experiment, regardless of some taking five minutes to reach orgasm while others needed as long as twenty.

It's no wonder it's important for a woman's mind to be totally free of any of the usual thoughts—mostly about work-related or domestic issues—racing through her mind and competing with those areas of the brain that should be left free to enjoy and develop the sexual impulses. Her mind needs to be free of these thoughts, if she is going to achieve the best orgasms possible.

Dr. Komisaruk stated, "In women, orgasm produces a very extensive response across the brain and the body. The evidence is that women tend to have longer orgasms and can experience several in rapid succession." A woman's orgasm lasts an average of ten to fifteen seconds, while a man's is thought to last for six. He also observed some women were able to 'think' themselves to orgasm, without any touching.

You can read a more comprehensive article on Dr. Komisaruk and his team's work here: http://www.nj.com/insidejersey/index. ssf/2010/04/science_consciousness_ and_the.html

Just one more piece of medical physiology, before we get on to some of the things we can consider when seeking a remedy for a low libido—your autonomic nervous system (ANS). This is part of the peripheral nervous system that controls involuntary actions, like heartbeat, breathing, digestion, and the widening or narrowing of your blood vessels.

It is the ANS that kicks in the spasms of orgasm and ejaculation in men. Incidentally, it is probably also responsible for a man's nocturnal erections.

Menopause

As with erectile dysfunction in men, there is a surfeit of information on menopause in women. It is only given a mention here because it is often identified as being the cause of a reducing, or even total loss of, interest in sex.

To write comprehensively about the probable or possible effects on your love life would require another book—so I'm not going there. If you feel your life is being negatively affected by menopause, please consult your doctor. There are medications that can help with your specific needs. The menopausal effect is different for every woman, but there are a few facts common to all I'll mention here.

Menopause is the end of menstruation for women. This means a woman's ovaries stop producing an egg every four weeks. Her monthly periods cease, and she will no longer be able to conceive. Having said that, because a woman's body could still be producing eggs but just very sporadically during perimenopause, conception does happen. It would be wise to continue using contraception methods for two years after your last period.

The average age (in the UK) for a woman to reach the menopause is 52, although it can be experienced by women in their 30s and 40s. Experienced at less than 45 years of age, this is referred to as premature menopause.

Menstruation, your monthly periods, can sometimes stop suddenly, but most women experience less frequency of periods, with longer intervals between each one, before they stop altogether.

The Causes of Menopause

It is inevitable, and it does affect every woman. It is caused by a change in the balance of the body's sex hormones. In the lead up to the menopause, estrogen levels decrease, which causes the ovaries to stop producing an egg each month. Estrogen is the female sex hormone that regulates a woman's periods.

Many women sail through menopause without a hint of trouble, while others suffer, to a greater or lesser degree, from the falling levels of estrogen. This can cause physical and emotional symptoms, including:

- Hot flushes

- Night sweats

- Mood swings

- Vaginal dryness

One 'old wives' tale' you can dismiss is you are going to put on weight. Middle-age spread is often blamed on the hormonal changes of menopause, but there is no proof of this. More likely weight gain is part of growing older and being less active—sorry about that.

Another common myth regarding menopause is if your mother had a difficult time going through menopause, you will too. Not true! There is no evidence to support such thinking. However, because the age at which menopause starts tends to be similar in mothers and daughters, this could give you an idea as to when you might expect yours to begin.[145;146].

Raising Your Libido

Now that we know what goes on, or what should go on, and where it stems from, we can begin to look at some of the more common reasons for a lack of libido. Unless there is an underlying medical reason (it is always a good idea to get a check-up and rule out a medical problem), there are a great many areas of our lives worth looking at to see if we can help ourselves in reaching our sexual goals.

Age

Remember, as we age our levels of testosterone—in women as well as men—reduce. This is not to say we should expect our sex drive to take a dive when we hit 50 or 60. Just keep in mind that with old age comes varying degrees of frailty, so don't expect sexual gymnastics in the bedroom when you're 80!

With advancing years comes greater sophistication, the application of a little more imagination and, greatest of all, patience, love and understanding. There is no reason to think all sex ends in the autumn of your years. There are folks who still enjoy sex well into their 80s, although maybe not every day.

It is my belief by staying sexually active you actually extend your life expectancy. There are so many hormones transported into tissue fluids and body cells, designed to provide energy, warmth, cell growth, and general fitness, produced in generous amounts naturally by the brain and body during sexual arousal and orgasm. This is not to be ignored in the greater picture of an extended life. Coupled with a healthy diet, a healthy weight and regular exercise, sex completes the picture of a healthy individual throughout his or her life. Of course, all those precedents to sex make serious, as well as necessary, contributions to an active and enjoyable sex life.[147]

Stress

Stress, and working too hard or for too long each day, can be the culprit of many problems. ED treatments can't do much if you are constantly exhausted, or not getting enough sleep—especially if these issues cause tension in your relationship. Write down what causes your stress and think about ways you can tackle them. Talk it over with your partner (see the chapter on "Communication"). Take time to relax and make an effort to share something you both enjoy doing at least once a week.

Dr. Carmine Pariante, a professor of biological psychiatry at King's College, London, stated "Give yourself a break; high stress levels can increase the hormone cortisol. Cortisol not only impairs the development of new brain cells but also your ability to cope with life's challenges. Taking a break can also help raise your libido; high levels of stress hormones have been shown to lower libido in women as well as men because the body focuses on producing cortisol instead of testosterone."[148]

It's worth mentioning here many women say stress is not their major issue. Instead, they feel depressed and frustrated their libido is not in sync with their partner. To be fair, men also express similar frustration. Talk it over with each other.

Sleep

Sleep, or rather the lack of it, can negatively affect your libido. Without a good night's sleep, your body is zapped of its available energy, and sex is no longer a priority. If you are struggling with this situation, try a gentle exercise program in the evening. Yoga or tai chi are good examples. Try the Lover's Steeple I described earlier. None of these are exhausting, and help relax the mind. Incidentally, yoga is also said to strengthen the pelvic floor muscles—another reason to take it up!

The Pill

According to Paul Carter, a consultant obstetrician and gynecologist at the 92 Harley Street Clinic in London, it's thought that by preventing ovulation, the pill also lowers levels of testosterone, the hormone responsible for sex drive. It also raises levels of the sex hormone binding globulin, which binds with testosterone and blocks its effects.

A woman's libido follows her monthly cycle. It goes up during ovulation, when estrogen is produced—and down after ovulation when progesterone is produced.

Sexually Transmitted Infections (STIs)/ Sexually Transmitted Diseases (STDs)

This is a subject that is well documented, and there are plenty of sources for information. For this reason, it is not my intention to cover the subject in this book. However, it is worth taking note, because STIs/STDs are the source of many problems, for many people, especially for the single and younger generations.

Some of the most common STIs/STDs are:

- Chlamydia
- Gonorrhoea
- Syphilis
- HIV
- Human Papilloma Virus (HVP)
- Herpes (HSV)

Chlamydia

Chlamydia infects the urethra in men and the cervix in women. People suffering from chlamydia often don't have symptoms for weeks, months or even years. For this reason, you can be infected and be totally unaware, and it is easily contracted. When you do have symptoms, they can include pain during sex and discharge from the penis or vagina. Luckily, chlamydia is a curable disease, plus using latex condoms are very effective at preventing the spread of this disease.

Gonorrhea

Gonorrhea, also known as "the clap," infects the same organs as chlamydia. Just like chlamydia, it may take awhile for symptoms to appear, once infected. Once symptoms occur, they include: burning during urination, and a white, yellow or green discharge from the penis. In the United States alone, there are 700,000 new cases of gonorrhea each year. Gonorrhea is not only transmitted by vaginal intercourse, but can be transmitted during oral sex, infecting the throat, as well. The Gonorrhea bacteria are easily treated with antibiotics, but these bacteria are constantly evolving, so new antibiotics have to be developed all the time.

As I write, the latest news is that a new strain of the bacterium has been discovered in North America that is immune to all known antibiotics. It is thought this new strain will have traveled to Europe by 2015. Let's hope the medical scientists come up with the answer very soon.

Syphilis

Syphilis was thought to be totally eradicated in the Western World until just a few years ago. With global travel becoming increasingly available, this STD has made a come-back, and the number of infections is growing. Caused by the bacteria *Treponema pallidum,* syphilis is transmitted by contact with syphilis sores. These can be located on the external portions of the genitals, the mouth, in the vagina, and in the rectum. Since some of these areas are not covered by a condom, condoms only offer some protection to the spread of this disease.

HIV/AIDS

HIV/AIDS was once only a STD exclusive to the gay fraternity. Not anymore. The number of infected persons is equally divided amongst all the sexual groupings. It is transmitted by the exchange of bodily fluid—semen, vaginal secretions, blood, and breast milk.

Human Papilloma Virus (HPV)

HPV is possibly the most common STD. A study performed in 1997 estimated that three-quarters of sexually active people has had HPV at one point in time. In 2007, another piece of research showed that nearly one-fourth of women are infected at any given time. Although some forms of HPV are linked to cervical cancer, other types can cause genital warts and others cause no symptoms at all.

Herpes (HSV)

Herpes is a viral STD. HSV1's most common symptom is cold sores. HSV2 is most often associated with genital sores. However, both forms are transmitted from mouth to genitals and vice versa. Herpes can be transmitted even when the infected person is symptom free. Although condoms can help reduce the risk of spreading herpes, they are not 100% effective.

If you have casual sex—as opposed to monogamous sex with a long-term partner—and you have not used a condom on every occasion, get down to a sexual health clinic and have a check-up. You owe it to yourself and those you have had sex with or have sex with in the future.

The point to make here is that many of these STIs/STDs, including the relatively minor ones like genital warts, can be avoided or minimized by using a condom. ALWAYS—and that includes ALL sexual activities, whether vaginal, penile, anal, or oral—wear a condom or have your partner wear a condom.

—— 24 ——

Quotes on Marriage by Famous Folk

The following is a lighthearted look at marriage, through the quotes from some famous people, over the years. Obviously, I don't necessarily personally agree with some of these quotes. However, I hope they give you a chuckle, as we end this book.

Enjoy!

"Don't worry about avoiding temptation. As you grow older, it will avoid you."

~ Winston Chuchill.

"Men marry because they are tired; women because they are curious.

Both are disappointed."

~ Oscar Wilde

"There's only one way to have a happy marriage and as soon as I learn what it is, I'll get married again."

~ Clint Eastwood

"Only two things are necessary to keep one's wife happy. First, let her think she's having her own way. And, second, let her have it."

~ Lyndon B Johnson

"Men who have a pierced ear are better prepared for marriage. They have experienced pain and bought jewelery."

~ Rita Rudner

"The most happy marriage I can imagine to myself would be the union of a deaf man to a blind woman."

~ Samuel Taylor Coleridge

"Marriage has many pains, but celibacy has no pleasure."

~ Samuel Johnson

"Remember that you're marrying a beautiful man you are in love with, and remember to make time for him, because I didn't."

~ Sarah Ferguson, Duchess of York

"Let him know you're happy: I smile whenever I see him. He always knows how thrilled I am that he's there with me."

~ Melanie Griffith

"Really, really good sex. I'm really good at it. Also, we talk a lot. Sometimes people hear us talking and think we 'over-talk' situations, but communication is everything."

~ Will Smith

"The husband who wants a happy marriage should learn to keep his mouth shut and his checkbook open."

~ Groucho Marx

"Be kind to each other. A lot of times we are nicer to strangers than the people that are close to us."

~ Michael Douglas

"Marriage is a series of desperate arguments people feel passionately about."

~ Katherine Hepburn

"I like having some mystery in our relationship. I like not knowing everything about my husband. I think it's good to have privacy and some secrets in our lives."

~ Sarah Jessica Parker

"Why does a woman work ten years to change a man's habits and then complain that he's not the man she married?"

~ Barbra Streisand

"I suppose it's about keeping love alive, learning how to fall in love over and over again, not taking each other for granted. Forgiveness and trust."

~ Patrick Swayze

"For marriage to be a success, every woman and every man should have their own bathroom."

~ Catherine Zeta-Jones

"A man doesn't know what happiness is until he's married. By then it's too late."

~ Frank Sinatra

"You need to be silly in a marriage, because it means you are not pretending. You're really being yourself."

~ Candace Bushnell (author of *Sex And The City*)

"You have to keep marriage alive; spice it up. I like to cook naked."

~ Christina Aguilera

Remember:

"Love can be wonderful, it can be difficult, it can be heart breaking, it can tear you apart, or it can be joyous and the making of you. But, in my opinion, the most important element, after trust, is communication. Never stop sharing your deepest thoughts, desires, emotions. Learn about each other's desires, needs, strengths and weaknesses—and learn to love them all. If this is not possible, it is unlikely you will survive very long as a couple."

~ *a final, serious, note from Clive Peters.*

List of Tables

List of Figures

Index

progesterone, 85, 87, 105, 305

progestin, 272-74

serotonin, 78, 81, 91, 203, 280

testosterone, See testosterone

circumcision, 12, 19

climax, 32, 34, 52, 83, 85, 104, 107-9, 126, 128, 168, 191, 224-25, 255, 266, 270

clitoris—

    anatomy of, 17-19

    location of, 18

    stimulation of, 118, 119, 123, 151, 156, 166, 168, 169, 172, 188, 190, 220, 224, 230, 231

    cock ring, 39, 41-2

contraception—

    female barrier methods, 274-75

    hormonal methods, 272-73

    IUD, 272, 273-74

    male condoms, 4, 5, 32, 128, 206-7, 215. 216, 218, 225, 226-27, 269-70, 276, 282, 306, 307

    oral, 5, 97, 267

    rhythm method, 271

    surgical methods, 271-72

    withdrawal, 270-71

corpora cavernosa, 14, 18

corpus spongiosum, 14, 18

cowper's gland, 14, 114, 149

cunnilingus. See oral sex

cystitis, 105, 221, 279-80, 283, 285, 286

E

edging, 33-35

ejaculate (female), 107-8, 112, 114-15

ejaculate (male)—

    composition, 82, 83

    increase the volume, 25, 44

    production of, 14-15, 71, 85

    retrograde, 164

    taste, 198-99

endorphins, 80-81, 90, 103, 258

epididymis, 13

erectile dysfunction—

    causes, 92, 100, 291

    description, 36

    injections, 39

    pellets, 39

    prescription treatment, 38

    statistics, 32, 36, 92

    supplements, 38, 96

erections—

    mechanics, 15-16

    quality, 26, 35-36, 37, 38

erogenous zones—

Endnotes

1 Hagan, P. (2011, March 15). Latest from the University of the Bleedin' Obvious: Couples stay together because women want love and men like sex | Mail Online. *Mail Online*. Retrieved July 31, 2013, from http://www.dailymail.co.uk/femail/article-1366314/Latest-University-Bleedin-Obvious-Couples-stay-women-want-love-men-like-sex.html

2 ibid

3 ibid

4 Alfred Kinsey, The Kinsey Institute

5 Kylstra, C. (n.d.). What women think of penises—Women sexual desires—Cosmopolitan. *Cosmopolitan*. Retrieved August 28, 2013, from http://www.cosmopolitan.com/cosmo-for-guys/sex-dating/what-she-thinks-when-she-first-sees-your-penis

6 ibid

7 ibid

8 MF Editors. (n.d.). What women think of male genitals—Penis women like—How to get the perfect penis—Men's Fitness. *Men's Fitness*. Retrieved August 28, 2013, from http://www.mensfitness.com/women/sex-tips/10-things-she%E2%80%99s-secretly-thinking-about-your-penis

9 Kylstra (n.d.)

10 MF Editors (n.d.)

11 ibid

12 Beland, N. (2008, September 15). What she thinks when she sees your package: Your most treasured organ, from a

woman's perspective. *Men's Health Magazine.* Retrieved August 28, 2013, from www.menshealth.com/sex-women/her-thoughts-your-penis

13 Kylstra (n.d.)

14 World map of the penis size worldwide by country. (n.d.). *TargetMap.* Retrieved August 28, 2013, from http://www.targetmap.com/viewer.aspx?reportId=3073

15 ibid

16 Opie, C., Atkinson, Q., Dunbar, R.I.M., Shultz, S. (2013). Male infanticide leads to social monogamy in primates. *Proceedings of the National Academy of Sciences*, eScholarID:203173

17 Seven-year itch is a myth—a marriage goes stale after ten years and 11 months | Mail Online. (2010, October 26). *Daily Mail.* Retrieved June 24, 2013, from http://www.dailymail.co.uk/news/article-1323722/Seven-year-itch-myth—marriage—goes-stale-years-11-months.html

18 Winkelmann RK (1959). "The erogenous zones: their nerve supply and significance". *Mayo Clin Proc* 34 (2): 39-47.

19 http://www.007b.com/breastfeeding_sexual.php

20 http://www.007b.com/breast_gallery.php

21 Stephenson, J. (2009). *Letting go of the glitz: the true story of one woman's struggle to live the simple life in Chelsea.* Bancyfelin: Crown House.

22 YouMagSocial, (2012, July 8) as a supplement to Mail on Sunday, Associated Newspapers, 2 Derry Street, London, W8 5TS.

23 Burchill, J. (2012, January 29). Spare me from the whining women who are giving feminism a bad name. *The Guardian.* Retrieved September 4, 2013, from http://www.theguardian.com/commentisfree/2012/jan/29/julie-burchill-female-friendship-feminism

24 Stephenson. (2009).

25   Why do blondes have a higher hair density than redheads?. (n.d.). *Hairfinder.com*. Retrieved September 5, 2013, from http://www.hairfinder.com/hairquestions/density.htm

26   Dean, I., & Siva-Jothy, M. (2011, December 14). Human fine body hair enhances ectoparasite detection. *Biology Letters*. Retrieved November 18, 2012, from http://rsbl.royalsocietypublishing. org/content/early/2011/12/08/rsbl.2011.0987.full.h tml

27   Fetish. (2013). *Merriam-Webster Online*. Retrieved September 5, 2013, from http://www.merriam-webster.com/dictionary/ fetish

28   Howorth, C. (2010, September 20). Merkins: Hollywood's Most Private Accessory. *The Daily Beast*. Retrieved September 5, 2013, from http://www.thedailybeast.com/articles/2010/09/20/ merkins-hollywoods-most-private-accessory.html

29   Cockerton, P. (2012, May 4). This Morning guest with hairy armpits shows off her body hair after 18 months of not shaving. *Mirror Online*. Retrieved September 5, 2013, from http://www.mirror.co.uk/news/real-life-stories/ this-morning-guest-with—hairy-armpits-shows-818470

30   Peters, C. (2013, March 24). Shaving—for women. *How to Maximize Your Manhood*. Retrieved September 5, 2013, from http://maximizeyourmanhood.wordpress.com/2013/03/24/ shaving-for-women/

31   Study confirms exercise-induced orgasm. (2012, March 19). *IU News Room: Indiana University*. Retrieved September 5, 2013, from http://newsinfo.iu.edu/news/page/normal/21547.html

32   Sukel, K. (2012, April 25). Is the BIG O all in your mind? Why everything you thought you knew about female sexuality is wrong. *Mail Online*. Retrieved September 5, 2013, from http://www.dailymail.co.uk/femail/article-2135138/Is—BIG-O-mind-Why-thought-knew-female-sexuality-wrong.html

33   Gray, R. (2013, February 10). Secrets of lasting love are hidden inside the brain say scientists. *Telegraph.co.uk*. Retrieved September 9, 2013, from http://www.telegraph.co.uk/

science/9859520/Secrets-of-lasting-love-are-hidden—inside-the-brain-say-scientists.html

34   ibid.

35   ibid

36   *Cephalalgia* the journal of the International Headache Society

37   ibid.

38   Charnetski, C., & Brennan, F. (Jun 2004). Sexual frequency and salivary immunoglobulin A (IgA). *Psychological Reports, 94*(3 (part 1)), 839-44.

39   Transcript taken from UK TV's Channel 4 program, *Embarrassing Bodies: Live from the Clinic,* Series 3, Episode 7 broadcast date June 4th, 2013.

40   ibid.

41   ibid.

42   ibid.

43   ibid.

44   ibid.

45   Carey, T. (2012, April 17). How fast is your body? SPERM. *Daily Mail*.

46   Vitamin D Increases Speed of Sperm Cells, Researchers Discover. (2011, May 25). *Science Daily*. Retrieved September 9, 2013, from www.sciencedaily.com/releases/2011/05/110525110157.htm.

47   Lerchbaum, Elisabeth at the Medical University of Graz, Austria, and studies published in *European Journal of Endocrinology*

48   ibid

49   Smith, G., Frankel, S., & Yarnell, J. (1997, December 20). Sex and death: are they related? Findings from the Caerphilly cohort study. *British Medical Journal*. Retrieved September 9, 2013, from http://www.bmj.com/content/315/7123/1641

50   Increasing Fertility Threefold. (2010, July 1). *American Friends of Tel Aviv University: Home Page*. Retrieved

September 9, 2013, from http://www.aftau.org/site/
News2?page=NewsArticle&id=12457

51   ibid.

52   What are the key statistics about prostate cancer?. (2013, May
     15). *American Cancer Society | Information and Resources for
     Cancer: Breast, Colon, Lung, Prostate, Skin.* Retrieved June
     21, 2013, from http://www.cancer.org/cancer/prostatecancer/
     detailedguide/prostate-cancer-key—statistics

53   Prostate cancer Key Facts : Cancer Research UK. (2013, January
     14). *Cancer Research UK: the UK's leading cancer charity :
     Cancer Research UK.* Retrieved June 21, 2013, from http://
     www.cancerresearchuk.org/cancer—info/cancerstats/keyfacts/
     prostate-cancer/cancerstats-key-facts-on-prostate-cancer

54   Fernandez, E. (2013, June 7). Men With Prostate Cancer
     Should Eat Healthy Vegetable Fats. *UCSF Helen Diller Family
     Comprehensive Cancer Center.* Retrieved September 9, 2013,
     from http://cancer.ucsf.edu/news/2013/06/07/men-with-
     prostate-cancer-should-eat-healthy-vegetable-fats.4710

55   ibid.

56   ibid.

57   ibid.

58   UK national newspaper and online news journal June 2013

59   Schneider, J. (2006). Metabolic And Hormonal Control Of The
     Desire For Food And Sex: Implications For Obesity And Eating
     Disorders. *Hormones and Behavior, 50*(4), 562-571.

60   Hodgekiss, A. (2011, March 29). Tonic water, white bread,
     painkillers—the unlikely passion killers sapping your sex
     drive. *Daily Mail.* Retrieved September 13, 2009, from www.
     dailymail.co.uk/health/article-1370939/Tonic-water-white-
     bread—painkillers—unlikely-passion-killers-sapping-sex-
     drive.html

61   Where did the "honeymoon" come from?. (n.d.). *Big Site
     of Amazing Facts.* Retrieved June 21, 2013, from www.

bigsiteofamazingfacts.com/where-did-the—honeymoon-come-from-and-how-did-the-word-honeymoon-originate

62   Mondaini, N., Cai, T., Gontero, P., Gavazzi, A., Lombardi, G., Boddi, V., et al. (2009). Regular Moderate Intake Of Red Wine Is Linked To A Better Women's Sexual Health. *Journal of Sexual Medicine*, *6*(10), 2772-7.

63   Virtue, D. (1995). *Constant craving: what your food cravings mean and how to overcome them.* Carson, CA: Hay House.

64   Saffron and ginseng 'shown to boost sexual desire'. (2011, March 28). *Telegraph.co.uk.* Retrieved September 10, 2013, from http://www.telegraph.co.uk/science/8411227/Saffron-and-ginseng-shown-to-boost-sexual-desire.html

65   Hodgekiss (2011).

66   ibid.

67   ibid

68   ibid

69   *Embarrassing Bodies.* (2013)

70   A Woman's Guide to Reviving Sex Drive. (2009, August 26). *WebMD.* Retrieved September 10, 2013, from http://www.webmd.com/sex-relationships/features/sex-drive-and-menopause?page=3

71   Lycopene. (2010, May 13). *American Cancer Society | Information and Resources for Cancer: Breast, Colon, Lung, Prostate, Skin.* Retrieved June 21, 2013, from www.cancer.org/treatment/treatmentsandsideeffects/complementaryandalternativemedicine/dietandnutrition/lycopene

72   Tomatoes: One of the World's Healthiest Foods. (n.d.). *TomatoWellness.com.* Retrieved September 10, 2013, from http://www.tomatowellness.com/health/tomato-are-healthy

73   Fenugreek can spice up things in the bedroom!. (2013, April 2). *Mid-Day.* Retrieved September 10, 2013, from http://www.mid-day.com/relationships/2013/apr/020413-fenugreek-aphrodisiac-boosts-sex-life-sex-and-relationships.htm

74   ibid.

75   ibid.

76   Choi, Y., C. Park, J. Jang, S. Kim, H. Jeon, W. Kim, S. Lee, and W. Chung. "Effects of Korean ginseng berry extract on sexual function in men with erectile dysfunction: a multicenter, placebo-controlled, double-blind clinical study." *International Journal of Impotence Research* 25.2 (2013): 45-50. Print.

77   ibid.

78   Hodgekiss (2011).

79   Morris, R. (2012, April 13). Solve his sex woes. *Cosmopolitan*. Retrieved September 20, 2013, from http://www.cosmopolitan.co.uk/_mobile/love-sex/tips/solve-his-sex-woes-men?ignoreCache=1

80   Barbara Bartlik, MD—Healthy Life Style Choices. (n.d.). *Barbara Bartlik, MD—Healthy Life Style Choices*. Retrieved September 20, 2013, from http://www.drbarbaramd.com/index.html

81   Evans, Randolph W. & Couch, R. (2001). "Orgasm and Migraine." *Headache: The Journal of Head and Face Pain* 111 (6), 512-514.

82   Altman, M. (2010, April 20). Rutgers lab studies female orgasm through brain imaging | NJ.com. *NJ.com*. Retrieved July 11, 2013, from http://www.nj.com/insidejersey/index.ssf/2010/04/science_consciousness_and_the.h tml

83   Sukel, K. (2012). *Dirty minds: how our brains influence love, sex, and relationships*. New York: Free Press.

84   ibid

85   Sexy Neuroscience. (2011, May 23). *The Connectome*. Retrieved September 20, 2013, from http://theconnectome.wordpress.com/2011/05/23/sexy-neuroscience/

86   2012 Great Male Survey Results. (2012, July 24). *AskMen*. Retrieved September 26, 2013, from http://www.askmen.com/specials/2012_great_male_survey/

87 Results From The 2013 Great Male Survey. (n.d.). *AskMen.* Retrieved September 26, 2013, from http://www.askmen. com/top_10/entertainment/results-from-the-2013-great-male-survey.html

88 Pappas, S. (2010, November 11). Study: Men Fake Orgasm, Too | LiveScience. *Science News.* Retrieved August 21, 2013, from http://www.livescience.com/8919—study-men-fake-orgasm. html

89 Moll Anderson Interviews Dr. Abraham Morgentaler— YouTube. (n.d.). *YouTube.* Retrieved August 15, 2013, from http://www.youtube.com/watch?v=s-6cGzOT0Vw

90 ibid

91 Kruger, D., & Hughes, S. (2011). Tendencies to fall asleep first after sex are associated with greater partner desires for bonding and affection. *Journal of Social, Evolutionary, and Cultural Psychology,* 5(4), 239-247.

92 ibid

93 Wilkes, D. (2011, August 17). Half of men know Miss Right after one date . . . but women need at least six. *Daily Mail.* Retrieved September 27, 2013, from http://www.dailymail. co.uk/femail/article-2026636/Half-men-know-Miss-Right—date—women-need-six.html

94 ibid

95 Lloyd, R. (2009, February 13). Saliva: Secret Ingredient in the Best Kisses. *LiveScience.com.* Retrieved October 30, 2013, from http://www.livescience.com/3328-saliva-secret-ingredient-kisses.html

96 Hendrie, C., & Brewer, G. (2009). Kissing As An Evolutionary Adaptation To Protect Against Human Cytomegalovirus-like Teratogenesis. *Medical Hypotheses, 74,* 222-224.

97 Frankel, V. (2008, December 11). More sex, less stress. *msnbc. com.* Retrieved October 30, 2013, from http://www.nbcnews. com/id/28146086/#.UnG9dBCMErc

98   Kirshenbaum, S. (2011, March 19). 20 Things You Didn't Know About . . . Kissing. *Discover Magazine*. Retrieved October 30, 2013, from http://discovermagazine.com/2011/jan-feb/20-things-you-didnt-know-about—kissing#.UnG-JBCMErc

99   Pelling, R. (2010, December 13). The secret of good kissing? Treat it like dancing . . . and follow your partner!. *Mail Online*. Retrieved October 30, 2013, from http://www.dailymail.co.uk/femail/article-1337984/Rowan-Pellings-sex-advice-The-secret-good-kissing-Treat-like-dancing—follow-partner.html

100   ibid

101   ibid

102   ibid

103   ibid

104   ibid

105   Khamsi, R. (2006, October 2). Women become sexually aroused as quickly as men. *NewScientist.com*. Retrieved November 17, 2013, from http://www.newscientist.com/article/dn10213-women-become-sexually-aroused-as—quickly-as-men.html#.UokeeOKMErc

106   Sex really does make men fall asleep. (2012, July 22). *The Telegraph*. Retrieved December 29, 2013, from http://www.telegraph.co.uk/health/healthnews/9418493/Sex-really-does-make-men-fall-asleep.html

107   ibid

108   ibid

109   Henderson, K. (n.d.). How To Have Anal Sex For The First Time. *YourTango*. Retrieved December 29, 2013, from http://www.yourtango.com/200681/anal-sex-for-beginners.html

110   ibid

111   ibid

112   ibid

113　Delvin, D. (n.d.). Anal sex. *Netdoctor*. Retrieved December 29, 2013, from http://www.netdoctor.co.uk/sexandrelationships/analsex.htm

114　Janssen, E. (n.d.). Special Reports—Why People Use Porn | American Porn | FRONTLINE |PBS. *PBS: Public Broadcasting Service*. Retrieved November 18, 2012, from http://www.pbs.org/wgbh/pages/frontline/shows/porn/special/why.html

115　History of Pornography. (n.d.). *History of Pornography*. Retrieved November 18, 2012, from http://www.pornographyhistory.com/

116　ibid

117　ibid

118　ibid

119　ibid

120　ibid

121　Statistics. (2010). *InternetSafety101.org*. Retrieved November 19, 2012, from http://www.internetsafety101.org/Pornographystatistics.htm

122　Stagger Statistics. (n.d.). *Mind Armor Training Tools*. Retrieved January 23, 2014, from http://www.mind-armor.com/staggering-statistics

123　Garver, L. (2006, April 26). Follow The Porn. *CBSNews*. Retrieved January 24, 2014, from http://www.cbsnews.com/news/follow-the-porn/

124　Blue, V. (2009, July 24). Are more women OK with watching porn?—CNN.com. *CNN.com*. Retrieved November 18, 2012, from http://www.cnn.com/2009/LIVING/personal/07/24/o.women.watching.porn/

125　ibid

126　Tall, S. (2010, March 25). In the Spotlight Anna Arrowsmith and Paul Walter. *Liberal Democrat Voice anna arrowsmith Tag*. Retrieved January 24, 2014, from http://www.libdemvoice.org/tag/anna-arrowsmith

127   Pornography Statistics. (n.d.). *Family Safe Media*. Retrieved November 18, 2012, from http://www.familysafemedia.com/pornography_statistics.html

128   Blue (2009)

129   Sinister power of the web—IOL SciTech | IOL.co.za. (2011, October 31). *IOL SciTech*. Retrieved December 11, 2012, from http://www.iol.co.za/scitech/technology/internet/sinister-power-of-the-web-1.1168074#.UMeD1HdACSo

130   Statistics. (2010).

131   Egypt moves to implement ban on online pornography | PRI. ORG. (2012, November 9). *PRI: Public Radio International*. Retrieved November 19, 2012, from http://www.pri.org/stories/world/middle-east/egypt-moves-to-implement-ban-on-online-pornography-12056.html

132   NuclearVacuum. (2010, July 14). File:Pornography laws. svg. *Wikipedia*. Retrieved November 19, 2012, from http://en.wikipedia.org/wiki/File:Pornography_laws.svg

133   What I Learned at Passages of Malibu and Candeocan.com About Porn Addiction | Porn Addiction Help. (n.d.). *Porn Addiction Help*. Retrieved December 11, 2012, from http://addictionporn.org/what-i-learned-at-passages-of-malibu-and-candeocan—com-about-porn-addiction/

134   Paraphilias. (2009, July 20). *Psychology Today: Health, Help, Happiness + Find a Therapist*. Retrieved December 21, 2012, from http://www.psychologytoday.com/conditions/paraphilias

135   Aggrawal, Anil (2009). *Forensic and Medico-legal Aspects of Sexual Crimes and Unusual Sexual Practices*. Boca Raton: CRC Press. pp. 369-82. ISBN 1-4200-4308-0.

136   Rex Ryan's Apparant Foot Fetish Not Necessarily Unhealthy—ABC News. (n.d.). *ABCNews.com—Breaking News, Latest News & Top Video News—ABC News*. Retrieved December 4, 2012, from http://abcnews.go.com/Health/rex-ryans-foot—video-not-necessarily-unhealthy/story?id=12467617#.UL5bNYZACSo

137 The Black Museum referred to was situated in the basements of the London Metropolitan Police Force HQ at Scotland Yard, Westminster, London. The premises have since moved to a new HQ. The Museum has never been open to the public and used for training purposes only. Nowadays the museum area is used primarily for lectures.

138 *Transcript extract from UK TV program shown on BBC1, 5 June 2011, entitled 'Inside The Human Body', written, produced and presented by Dr Michael Mosley.

139 Lambskin Condoms FAQ. (2012). *Lambskin Condoms FAQ*. Retrieved July 14, 2013, from http://lambskincondoms. org/#history

140 Birth Control and the Rhythm Method. (2013). *WebMD*. Retrieved July 14, 2013, from http://www.webmd.com/sex/ birth-control/rhythm-method

141 Have your hottest sex ever this winter :: Men's Health. (n.d.). *Men's Health Magazine*. Retrieved May 21, 2013, from http://www.menshealth.co.uk/sex/better/ have-your-hottest-sex-ever-this-winter-379088

142 O'Connor, A. (2006, July 18). The Claim: Chocolate Is an Aphrodisiac—New York Times. *The New York Times*. Retrieved May 21, 2013, from http://www.nytimes.com/2006/07/18/ health/18real.html?_r=0

143 What I need to know about Bladder Control for Women— National Kidney and Urologic Diseases Information Clearinghouse. (2012, June 29). *National Kidney and Urologic Diseases Information Clearinghouse*. Retrieved May 21, 2013, from http://kidney.niddk.nih.gov/kudiseases/pubs/bcw_ez/#ack

144 Black, T. (Director). (2012). *Hope springs* [Motion picture]. USA: Sony Pictures Home Entertainment.

145 Wilson, M.M. (1987). Menopause. Clin Geriatr Med, 19(3):483-506.

146   Sherwin, B.B. (1987). The role of androgen in the maintenance of sexual functioning in oophorectomized women. Psychosom Med, 49(4):397-409.

147   Doheny, K. (2013). 10 Surprising Health Benefits of Sex. *WebMD*. Retrieved May 22, 2013, from www.webmd.com/sex-relationships/guide/10-surprising-health—benefits-of-sex

148   Anacker, C. & Pariante, C. (2012) 'Stress and Neurogenesis Can adult neurogenesis buffer stress responses and depressive behaviour?' *Molecular Psychiatry,* 17(1), pp.9-10.

Lightning Source UK Ltd.
Milton Keynes UK
UKOW04f1641010714

234389UK00001B/12/P